SPEAKING IN TONGUES:
THE SONGS OF VAN MORRISON

By the same authors

Martin Buzacott

Fiction:
Charivari (Picador), *Narrenschiff* (Picador)

Non-fiction:
The Death of the Actor: Shakespeare on page and stage (Routledge)

Drama:
Kingaroy (Currency)

Andrew Ford

Non-fiction:
Composer to Composer: Conversations about contemporary music (Hale & Iremonger), *Illegal Harmonies: Music in the 20th century* (ABC Books), *Undue Noise: Words about music* (ABC Books)

CDs:
Whispers (Tall Poppies TP053), *Harbour* (TP128), *Icarus* (TP150)

SPEAKING IN TONGUES:
THE SONGS OF VAN MORRISON

MARTIN BUZACOTT
and
ANDREW FORD

ABC
Books

First published by ABC Books for the
AUSTRALIAN BROADCASTING CORPORATION
GPO Box 9994 Sydney NSW 2001

Copyright © Martin Buzacott and Andrew Ford 2005

First published in May 2005

All rights reserved. No part of this publication may be reproduced, stored in a retrieval system or transmitted in any form or by any means, electronic, mechanical, photocopying, recording or otherwise, without the prior written permission of the Australian Broadcasting Corporation.

National Library of Australia
Cataloguing-in-publication data:

Speaking in tongues: the songs of Van Morrison.

  Bibliography.
  Includes index.
  ISBN 0 7333 1297 7.

  1. Morrison, Van, 1945- — Criticism and interpretation. I. Australian Broadcasting Corporation. II. Title.

782.42164

Cover design by Fisheye Design
Typeset in 11/17pt Sabon by Kirby Jones
Printed and bound in Australia by Griffin Press, Adelaide

5 4 3 2 1

Oh journey-man, oh journey-man,
Before this endless belt began
Its cruel revolutions, you and she
Naked in Eden shook the apple tree.

Alun Lewis (1915–44)

I am of Ireland
And of the holy land
Of Ireland.
Good sir, pray I thee,
Of sainte charity
Come and dance with me
In Ireland.

Anon. (thirteenth century)

CONTENTS

Introduction *Van Morrison at a glance*	1
Part One	
A soul in wonder: Themes and variations	19
Childhood	21
Musical heroes	34
Transcendence and religion	50
Nature and literature	61
Complaints	73
Part Two	
A working man in his prime	85
Nothing but a stranger in this world (1968–1974)	87
Cry for home (1975–1991)	160
On with the show (1992–2003)	255
Epilogue	
Speaking in tongues: The voice of Van Morrison	305
Appendix 1 Discography	316
Appendix 2 Name-checks in Van Morrison's songs	339
Bibliography	344
Index	346
Acknowledgments	360

INTRODUCTION

VAN MORRISON AT A GLANCE

There is currently a website that describes itself as 'the Virtual Shrine to Gustav Mahler'. It is a mock-religious page on which music-lovers who had previously doubted the quality of the Viennese composer's works testify to a moment of enlightenment, when the wonders of the music and the genius of the composer were manifested in one blinding epiphany. In hundreds of such testimonies, the situation is always similar. Mahler's art, which had appeared self-important, long-winded, repetitive, contradictory and simply overrated to these web writers, suddenly revealed itself to be coherent, intensely beautiful, fanatically true to its own principles, and possessed of incomparable aesthetic power. The listener suddenly 'gets it', and the internal logic of the art exerts its spell. This occurs with particular intensity in the case of Mahler, but to a certain extent it is a scenario that is played

Introduction

out over and over again throughout the arts — where greatness in depth emerges from superficial inconsistency and where transcendental revelation is conveyed through facile expression.

In the blaring, heightened, hyper-commercial world of modern popular music, genius emerges routinely from the most humble and inauspicious surroundings. Drugged-out, drunken individuals with no musical training can produce songs that change the world. Singers who can't hold a tune can convey anthems that just don't sound as good when sung with 'proper' intonation and phrasing. And with appropriate twelve-bar backing, the most naturally inarticulate hooligan can become a poet whose words inspire a generation. Art, then, has the ability to transcend the individual whose name is associated with it, and its worth cannot adequately be judged by simple reference to the superficial means of its dissemination. This is never more so than in the case of Van Morrison.

One of the most distinctive singers in the history of popular music, over four decades the Belfast-born Morrison has written and sung songs of mystical power and reminiscence. They are comforting and thrilling by turns, dreadful sometimes, formulaic quite often, but as a totality they chart some of the most profound and sublime moments in the history of pop. And yet, as hundreds of interviewers have discovered to their exasperation and cost, the man himself is another matter altogether. At a time of life when middle-aged complacency might have beckoned, Morrison remains his truculent, uncommunicative self, unhelpful with the media, reluctant to explain many of his songs from an external perspective, and, if

Introduction

reports are to be believed, downright obnoxious at times in his dealings with colleagues in the industry. In other words, the gap between the man and his 'healing' music is more pronounced than with most other artists.

But as with the Mahler devotees, Morrison's fans understand the difference between superficial appearances and artistic truth. They are loyal and will forgive 'Van the Man' just about anything — which is helpful because over the years there has been plenty to forgive. There's his surly behaviour, onstage as well as off. There are the concerts where he'll race through the song list as though he deeply wishes he was somewhere else. There are his saxophone and harmonica solos that so often self-destruct. And there are albums that seem, at least on first hearing, to contain exactly the same tracks as their predecessors.

It's a significant list of grievances. On close analysis, however, these foibles lapse into near-irrelevance. Why should Van Morrison be pleasant to people? He's a singer, not a social worker. Why should he always enjoy live performance when so many of the great musicians of the twentieth century, including Glenn Gould and the Beatles, shared his antipathy to the stage? And why shouldn't he, if the mood strikes him, fumble around with instruments on which he is less than proficient? After all, absence of technical mastery is not necessarily a hindrance in expressing emotion through popular music.

In his songs, Morrison's personal preoccupations are revealed at exhaustive length, in riffs, themes, images and phrases that constantly recur on album after album. Any devotee can list the repetitions instantly: the slipstreams; the cool, clear crystal waters; the backstreet jellyroll; the viaducts

Introduction

and pylons; the reminiscences of a Northern Ireland childhood; the transcendental moments when time stands still; the search for quietness and an audience who will listen; the checklists of radio stations, rhythm-and-blues artists, literary and sporting heroes and other idols of his youth; the glorification of music as the source of adolescent identity.

These themes and variations proceed with remarkable consistency over four decades of work, but they exist only in relation to the voice that is singing them. And Morrison is fundamentally that — a voice. It is a voice of distinction, instantly recognisable, yet it is remarkably flexible and diverse in its expressiveness. To start with, there's Morrison the belter, his largish chest heaving for deep breath as he screams into 'Here Comes the Night' and other numbers that he first sang with Them in the mid 1960s. It's a bull's roar of a thing, a kind of refined primal scream. Or we have guttural Van, gruffly burbling his way through a whole concert, with little change in pitch except to express dissatisfaction, like some curmudgeonly old granddad whingeing about having to entertain the children on his own for an hour. Growling is another part of it. When combined, wordlessly, with heavy breathing, it becomes an extended 'harrumph' that can sustain entire songs.

At the opposite end of the vocal spectrum is the angelic falsetto, clear and pure, that we hear on 'Crazy Love' (from 1970's *Moondance* album) — Van in choirboy mode mixed with a dash of Smokey Robinson. It's a head voice that he sometimes adopts in combination with the guttural timbre, where the changes in style balance each other and create an entire world of sound; his only rival here is Tom Waits. Added

Introduction

to this are his distinctive whispers, wheeled out whenever he wishes to establish the intimate mood that has been such a feature of his work over the years. Variations on the whisper include hands placed over the microphone and 'singing' through the harmonica.

And of course there's the chat, too — Van not singing but talking, as he frequently does when he reminisces. Another vocal device is Sprechstimme, or 'speech-singing', a technique made famous in twentieth-century masterpieces such as Schoenberg's *Pierrot lunaire* but which Van has perfected in popular music. When it occurs, as it does in 'So Quiet in Here', a standout track from 1990's *Enlightenment*, it is as if Van, caught in the emotion of the moment and the world of the song, loses interest in singing, becoming preoccupied instead with an exploration of the feelings that he remembers now from a distant past, and only partially connecting with what may once have purported to be the actual tune at hand. And this is to say nothing of the keening — that extraordinary expression of Celtic grief which, if not literally employed as in the folk tradition, certainly imbues with its spirit almost everything Morrison sings. Like a thousand Irish bards before him, Morrison is a wailer for what has been lost.

The ancient Greek philosopher Archilochus's distinction between hedgehogs and foxes, popularised by Isaiah Berlin, is not unhelpful in a discussion of Morrison's art. The clever fox knows many things; the hedgehog knows one big thing. Musically speaking, Haydn, Stravinsky, Louis Armstrong, Benny Goodman, John Lennon and Elvis Costello are all foxes. Van Morrison, along with Mahler, Anton Bruckner, Olivier Messiaen, Thelonious Monk, Harrison Birtwistle and

Introduction

Bruce Springsteen, is avowedly a hedgehog. Throughout his work, one emotion fuels a multiplicity of stylistic shifts. But more than that, Van's work is a tissue of quotations and vaguely recalled influences. The name-checks of r&b, soul and jazz legends throughout his music are the external signs of a musical mind recalling the sounds that came together to form his mature personality. And within the music itself, the traces of past idols establish the very essence of each work's identity.

Increasingly, Morrison's live performances have tended to consist of medleys, one song clashing with or emerging from another. Just as Mahler juxtaposes offstage brass bands with syrupy onstage strings and twisted *ländlers* — the soundscape of his own youth — so Morrison forms new work from a combination of, say, 'Stormy Monday', 'Have You Ever Loved a Woman?' and 'No Rollin' Blues'. It's not so much an act of creation as a journey of remembrance. Morrison might write the same song over and over, but in performance he adds to it. He adds new layers, while stripping others away, obsessively exploring his musical world. Even a hedgehog, lying low to the ground and seeing only one thing, can capture the universe in a single glance.

Van was born George Ivan Morrison on 31 August 1945, the only child of Belfast shipyard worker George Morrison and his wife Violet. He grew up with an intense intellectual curiosity, but his overwhelming passion for music meant that he had left school by the age of fifteen and was already, to all intents and purposes, a professional musician. Although he lacked a formal education, the young Morrison possessed an

Introduction

encyclopedic knowledge of American popular music gained via pirate radio and his father's extensive record collection. He was also a voracious reader and — as several important song lyrics later testify — seems from an early age to have been interested in poetry and mysticism.

Having cut his musical teeth in Irish show bands and the fledgling Belfast r&b scene, the teenage Van toured Europe in various bands, the most notable of which was the Monarchs, playing to American servicemen and cutting long-forgotten records. But with the formation of Them in 1964, Morrison was on his way to international stardom. Having wished from the start to become merely a 'working musician', the unexpected fame hung heavily upon him and his discomfort with it would shape much of his subsequent (notoriously bad) social behaviour, and furnish many unfortunate song lyrics.

Them's 'Baby, Please Don't Go', 'Here Comes the Night' and 'Gloria' — the last two of which are still staples of Morrison's live sets — gave him international hits and the opportunity for serious exploitation by management. Multiple personnel changes in the band, extensive American touring and spectacular disputes over money led to Them's eventual disintegration, and by early 1967 the young and already-embittered Van had returned to his childhood home on Hyndford Street, East Belfast, to lick his wounds and record some demos of original material.

But later that year, American producer Bert Berns (with whom Them had worked with some success in London) extended an invitation for Van to come to New York to record for his label, Bang Records. The result was the hit 'Brown Eyed Girl'. Initially it wasn't enough to establish Van's solo career —

Introduction

and neither was the album *Blowin' Your Mind*, Bang's ill-advised attempt to milk what it could from this US chart success — but with an American partner (and subsequent wife) in Janet Planet, Van was soon back across the Atlantic with a new and highly original musical direction. Now signed to the prestigious Warner Bros. label, and determined not to be typecast any more as a rock star, he began to explore acoustic, folk and jazz styles, often simultaneously. One of the great pop albums was brewing.

Over just two main recording sessions in early autumn 1968 (an intervening session was aborted), a musical marvel emerged. Still a routine listing among the ten greatest albums of all time, *Astral Weeks* remains perhaps the key album in Morrison's catalogue, its first lines establishing a landscape that the artist would continue to roam for the next thirty-five years: 'If I ventured in the slipstream / Between the viaducts of your dream'.

Slipstreams and viaducts, dreams and backroads, and perhaps most importantly the desire to be born again: each idea would be revisited over and over, right down to the present day. The sound-world of *Astral Weeks*, however, was less easy to duplicate. The one-off combination of backing musicians included drummer Connie Kay from the Modern Jazz Quartet, ex–Miles Davis bassist Richard Davis, and flautist/saxophonist John Payne. Hardly speaking to each other, they found themselves improvising music with which they had little natural affinity, and yet creating an album whose magical sound and palpable atmosphere of creative inspiration still sounds immediate and fresh today. Not even the participants could ever fully re-create the magic — 'Slim

Introduction

Slow Slider' being the product of a soundcheck rather than the formal sessions — and only Kay would work again with Morrison on later projects. The resulting album offered up no singles, but continues to sell well, introducing each new generation of fans to a man who, aged just twenty-three at the time of the album's release in November 1968, sounds like a baccy-spitting, hard-bitten Delta blues legend.

Van and Janet moved to Woodstock in upstate New York, where the songs for the next record began to take shape. Released in early 1970 and titled *Moondance*, the feel was more commercial this time around, and the album contained several tracks that would become standards. The folk-rock lead-off track 'And It Stoned Me' recalls a fishing expedition the singer made as a twelve-year-old; the title track is now his most covered song and a little masterpiece of jazz-pop, while the powerful 'Caravan' still works wonders in live performance. Despite the collection's more poppy sentiments compared to *Astral Weeks* — a quality that resulted in 'Come Running' and 'Moondance' becoming modest hits — the critics reacted positively. Morrison's artistic and commercial status was assured.

As the 1970s proceeded, the wild oscillations of style and quality that we now recognise as a Morrison trademark began to appear. The r&b feel of 'Domino' and its parent album *His Band and the Street Choir* (released later in 1970) was followed by perhaps his most feeble work — notwithstanding the punchy hit single, 'Wild Night' — 1971's *Tupelo Honey*, in which too much time spent between Woodstock and California resulted in the worst of both musical worlds. In 1972, however, *Saint Dominic's Preview* represented a return to form, perhaps inspired (if that is the word) by the breakdown of his relationship with Janet Planet. If the epic, rip-your-heart-out 'Listen to the Lion' is anything to go by, the death-throes of his marriage increased Van's level of musical intensity. With its extraordinary range of vocalisations, improvisatory structure and worlds-apart feel, 'Listen to the Lion' is a strong contender for the definitive Van Morrison song. The album's other standout tracks included 'Jackie Wilson Said (I'm in Heaven When You Smile)' and the watershed 'Almost Independence Day'.

In 1973, *Hard Nose the Highway* brought with it new musical ambition and another monster of a song in 'Snow in San Anselmo'. That opening track's dramatic changes in tempo and style, boisterous choir, and the singular vocal incantation of 'my waitress, my waitress, my waitress' make it a Van special, which almost compensates for the same album's inclusion of a truly dreadful rendition of the Kermit the Frog song 'Bein' Green'. Touring material from these albums with the big-band sound of the Caledonia Soul Orchestra resulted in *It's Too Late to Stop Now* (1974), one of the great live albums of popular music history and proof that, for all his legendary disasters on stage, when he's in the mood Van Morrison is virtually incomparable.

A return to Ireland for a holiday, and an aesthetically fateful rental car journey through rural districts, changed Van's perspective, and in the misty, mystical *Veedon Fleece* he created an unmistakeably Irish-sounding album that was rock music's equivalent of the haunted ancient ruins of a lost civilisation. Initially difficult to comprehend when released in late 1974, and a disappointing seller compared with its

Introduction

predecessors, it was the first of Van's 'transcendental' albums, trying to connect with an idealised, mythical past.

Veedon Fleece introduced a particularly potent theme that would run through much of his subsequent work. Its modal, bardic echoes of some ancient wisdom can be felt in several albums from the 1980s, including *Common One* (1980), *A Sense of Wonder* (1984) and even the more commercially oriented *Avalon Sunset* (1989). But the African–American influence on Morrison's music didn't lose its grip entirely and the albums from the late 1970s included the funky but disappointing *A Period of Transition* (1977) — his first release after two-and-a-half years of apparent inactivity — and the Californian-sounding *Wavelength* (1978) and *Into the Music* (1979), the last of which was the true 'comeback' album for the Ulsterman.

As the 1980s dawned, God began to enter the scene. And healing too. Inspired by Cyril Scott's book *Music: Its Secret Influences Through the Ages* and countless other quasi-philosophical works, Morrison became fixated on the healing powers of his art, a fascination that would culminate explicitly in *The Healing Game* (1997). Alice Bailey's brand of Theosophy influenced *Beautiful Vision* (1982), while an interest in Scientology seems to have led to the 1983 release *Inarticulate Speech of the Heart*. Both these albums were well represented on another live collection, 1984's generally disappointing *Live at the Grand Opera House, Belfast*. But if God remained elusive, Morrison's continued searching produced glorious songs, such as 'A Sense of Wonder' and 'In the Garden', and two of his best albums — *No Guru, No Method, No Teacher* (1986) and *Poetic Champions Compose* (1987).

Introduction

In 1988, the influence of Irish folk music, which had permeated so much of Morrison's work thus far, was rendered with tremendous urgency in his famous collaboration with the Chieftains, *Irish Heartbeat*. Having spent so much time singing African–American music like an Irishman, now Van sang Irish music like an African–American, and the results were compelling. *Irish Heartbeat* introduced a legion of new fans to his music and 'explained' much about the man's music and music-making that had previously seemed enigmatic. When it came to the crunch, Van Morrison revealed himself as an authentic Irish artist whose career had forced him into a kind of musical exile.

Meanwhile the search for meaning in the past continued with more of his mystical quests for silence and a sense of spirituality in *Avalon Sunset*, 1990's *Enlightenment* and, the following year, *Hymns to the Silence*, a double album. *Too Long in Exile* (1993) had its moments but scarcely prepared the way for another fine live album, *A Night in San Francisco* (1994), with its breathtaking r&b takes on standards and Morrison originals alike.

Morrison had lived in America for many years following the slow-burning success of *Astral Weeks*, but during the late '70s he returned more and more to Britain, recording at Richard Branson's studios in Oxfordshire, buying property, and commuting back and forth across the Atlantic. Reflecting this change of focus, his subsequent musical output has tended to be more popular in the UK than in his previous 'market', America. In the 1980s, he became a British resident once more, living variously in London and Bath but progressively gravitating back to Ireland.

Introduction

Never comfortable in his relationship with the media, in the 1990s he became a sorry victim of the tabloids via his long-standing and unusually public relationship with former Miss Ireland and one-time Eurovision Song Contest compere Michelle Rocca. The couple appeared together at public events and even on stage (with Rocca reciting the words of W.B. Yeats and other Irish poets in Morrison's concerts), and the notoriously abrasive singer appeared genuinely in love with the beauty queen, sparking all manner of cruel commentary on their contrasting physical attributes. But with marriage rumours circulating, the gutter press revealed that Rocca had been two-timing Van with a prominent racing identity, and the ensuing relationship breakdown and public humiliation affected him deeply.

In the meantime, work drove him on. Throughout the 1990s and into the twenty-first century, Morrison has continued to expand his musical horizons, or at least to explore his obvious areas of influence in more depth, sometimes in partnership with collaborators. These partners have included jazz great Jimmy Witherspoon, soul man Ray Charles, and blues legends Junior Wells, B.B. King and, most important of all, John Lee Hooker. Van would also team up with the Chieftains on occasions as well as working with more middle-of-the-road artists like Cliff Richard, Tom Jones, Mark Knopfler and his daughter Shana Morrison. During the 1990s, Georgie Fame, a keyboard player who himself had enjoyed a short-lived stellar career as a solo artist in the 1960s, played a very significant role as Morrison's stage and studio sidekick.

In between by-now-typical Morrison-style albums such as *Days Like This* (1995), *The Healing Game* (1997), *Back on*

Introduction

Top (1999) and *Down the Road* (2002) were diversions into the music of his youth. Van went jazz on *How Long Has This Been Going On* (1995) and paid homage to Mose Allison on *Tell Me Something* (1996). He teamed up with his boyhood skiffle hero Lonnie Donegan on *The Skiffle Sessions* (2000), and made a curious digression into rockabilly on *You Win Again* (2000), his collaboration with Linda Gail Lewis. More recently he has explored the lounge-jazz and easy-listening side of his musical personality, in *What's Wrong With This Picture?* (2003).

And like so many legends before him, the Morrison vault has been trawled for unreleased tracks and alternative takes. The resultant *The Philosopher's Stone* (1998) is a double album with no particular musical direction, but is important for its inclusion of illuminating rejects like the complaint song 'Drumshanbo Hustle' and Morrison's singing Yeats's lyric 'Crazy Jane on God'.

As Morrison turns sixty, the pattern is well established: an album every year or so, the themes of childhood continuing, either explicitly in the lyrics or in the musical styles adopted and collaborators chosen. As this book goes to press, almost eighteen months have passed since his previous release. It's only a matter of time . . .

In spite of the singer's reluctance to assist his interpreters, the various biographies and studies of Van Morrison have remained fixated on the man behind the songs and have consistently sought to discover and reveal the 'word' of the creator. This trend towards seeking Morrison's own words as explanation began with writers Ritchie Yorke and Johnny

Introduction

Rogan in the 1970s, continued with John Collis, Brian Hinton and Steve Turner in the 1990s, and has carried over into the new millennium, with Clinton Heylin's recent biography structured entirely around direct quotes from Morrison and his colleagues. It seems the more obtuse and unhelpful Van becomes, the more determined his biographers are to seek him out as the point of origin for meaning in his music. But in the end, Morrison has demonstrated time and again that there is little that can genuinely be revealed about the music (or the man) that is not in the music already.

Speaking in Tongues: The Songs of Van Morrison is not a biography. As the title implies, this book focuses on the artist's words and music, and the relationship between them. Live albums will be referred to regularly, but the songs on the official studio albums (that is, excluding the hotchpotch *Blowin' Your Mind* and projects that Van has been involved in outside his solo releases) will form the subject for the main discussion. Of his collaborative projects, only *Irish Heartbeat* has been included among the twenty-six albums featured here, such is its importance in Morrison's work as a whole.

The songs are approached from two perspectives. Part One sets out the main themes and motifs that continue to underlie Van Morrison's work — recurrent ideas which surface in songs from all stages of his career. These themes and motifs furnish Morrison's personal intellectual lexicon and philosophical grammar: his dictionary of self-quotation in which lyrics in a song from, say, the 1990s, put themselves into 'dialogue' with others from the 1960s or 1970s.

Like Tennyson's Ulysses, Van Morrison is a part of all that he has met, a storehouse of experience and memory. To

Introduction

listen to him singing his songs is to get inside his cluttered mind and join him on remembered journeys around the East Belfast of his youth — up this street, down that avenue, across the viaducts, beneath the pylons. As in the 1982 track 'Cleaning Windows', you are carrying a window-cleaner's ladder, on your back a knapsack containing Paris buns, a Jimmie Rodgers record and a copy of Jack Kerouac's *The Dharma Bums*.

The landscape has a familiarity, and yet you feel a sense of wonder. All around you are childhood memories, and they provoke your imagination, inspiring you to the extent that you are constantly searching for a higher meaning and a connection with a perfect silence, most likely to be found in nature or in some ancient past.

Frequently disappointed in your quest, and too often encountering shysters and people who distract you or seek to thwart your progress, you soldier on out of a sense of duty and because it's your job (you are a Protestant and have a work ethic to match). Sometimes when you're in a good mood you might hanker after a companion who will share the mystical quest with you, and, if she's female, you'll walk with her down by the river (or railroad, or avenue), listening together to the wind in the willows. And at day's end the two of you might retire inside for a little bit of conversation, play some old blues, soul or jazz records, and then finish it off with that old backstreet jellyroll . . .

These repeated patterns of creative behaviour — the childhood reminiscences, the spiritual searching, the nature-worship, the homages to musical idols, the themes of innocence, experience and complaint — are everywhere in

Introduction

Morrison's work. They are the building blocks from which he constructs his songs and imaginative landscapes. So it's worth exploring each of the themes in some detail and comparing some of their more notable manifestations in classic songs such as 'Madame George' (from 1968's *Astral Weeks*), 'A Sense of Wonder' (*A Sense of Wonder*, 1984), 'In the Garden' (*No Guru, No Method, No Teacher*, 1986; *A Night in San Francisco*, 1994) and 'On Hyndford Street' (*Hymns to the Silence*, 1991), as well as many lesser-known tracks. Any such discussion will in part be arbitrary, and some crucial ideas — music as a healing force, for one — are better placed within the specific discussion of the individual albums, in Part Two.

True artistic expression doesn't take kindly to being pigeonholed, of course, and, as will become obvious in Part One, the five main themes of Van Morrison's songs are by no means stand-alone motifs. They are interrelated and synergistic. And in the case of Van Morrison — who has had one of the most consistent careers in popular music — most of them were there right from the very beginning.

The second part of this book traces these themes chronologically, album by album, from *Astral Weeks* in 1968 up to *What's Wrong With This Picture?*, his most recent release. So Part One is the 'harmony', in which Morrison's themes are elaborated, and Part Two is the 'melody' of his career, with the Epilogue concentrating on the 'means of production' — a final appraisal of that extraordinary instrument which is Van Morrison's voice.

PART ONE

A soul in wonder

THEMES AND VARIATIONS

CHILDHOOD

'The youth of a thousand summers' is a familiar figure in Van Morrison's songs and the desire to go back in time is a stock-in-trade. Virtually every album contains songs, or at least individual lyrics, in which childhood is evoked, often in rapt, mystical wonder. It's not the simple nostalgia of a middle-aged man. For Van Morrison, childhood is a state of being, a world of innocence and beauty which the contemporary world has abandoned.

In September and October 1968 when he recorded his first proper solo album, *Astral Weeks*, he had just turned twenty-three. Superficially the degree of retrospection embodied in it might seem surprising. Most 23-year-old men do not sing about their childhood, they don't even sing about the past. Most 23-year-old men sing about their girlfriends or their car, and the songs are in the present tense or in an ideal, chimerical future. But there, on *Astral Weeks*, on what are still regarded as some of his finest songs — 'Cyprus Avenue, 'Madame George' and the album's title track — Morrison is already busy reminiscing.

A soul in wonder

It's very easy to hear these early songs as naked autobiography, which in part they are, but at a deeper level, they look beyond, to a world not so much of memory but of imagination in which the actual locations of the material world are transformed into exemplars of a spiritual state.

In the first verse of the first song — 'Astral Weeks' itself — we hear about venturing in 'the slipstream' that is 'between the viaducts of your dream', and we encounter his desire to be 'born again'. These are words, images and themes that Morrison revisits to this day, and from the start some of these were more transparent in their meaning than others. The viaduct, for instance, appears to be a tangible symbol of his childhood and early teenage years in East Belfast, much like the 'pylons' referred to at the end of his 1979 album *Into the Music* and many times since. One imagines these viaducts and pylons as a vivid setting for the young Van's activities: tadpoles in jam-jars, illicit cigarettes, r&b records and the first, furtive fumblings of adolescent sex.

From the very start of his solo singing career, it was these songs in celebration of an idyllic youth that were least close to jazz, blues, soul or gospel — the popular music forms in which Morrison had been steeped as a child. Harmonically, these and all the childhood songs that followed tend to have a modal simplicity whose roots are in Celtic folk song.

'Astral Weeks', 'Cyprus Avenue' and 'Madame George' relate to Belfast (in so far as Cyprus Avenue is in Belfast and Madame George herself is in Cyprus Avenue), but to suggest that they are a slice of daily life from Morrison's childhood would be overly simple. The lyrics, as celebrated rock scribe

Greil Marcus suggested, display the influence of Bob Dylan in their apparent tendency to associate freely.

'Cyprus Avenue' sets out simply enough with a few strummed chords on acoustic guitar, but then a harpsichord appears, playing the riff that will colour the entire song. Harpsichords in pop music were certainly not unprecedented in 1968, but they were rare. The acoustic bass line grows more elaborate as the song continues, and other instruments, notably a flute and a violin, contribute phrases of ever-increasing intensity and melodic spontaneity. But it is Morrison's words and his voice that make the song compelling. The singer is trapped. He is 'caught . . . on Cyprus Avenue', 'conquered in a car seat', his 'tongue gets tied', and there's 'nothing' he can do. And we hear the frustration in Morrison's vocals, particularly in the tongue-tied stammering.

The 'mansion on the hill' that provokes this state of near-paralysis is possibly a girls' school and its teenage occupants, and as the song gains momentum, the acoustic guitar strumming more boldly and rhythmically, swelling strings filling out the texture, so Morrison's voice alters. The repetitions are no longer a speech impediment but an outpouring of ecstasy: 'No, no, no, nobody stops me from loving you,' he sings. The next lines ('So young and bold / Fourteen years old') are probably addressed to the girl in question, but they might equally well describe the singer of the song, finally conquering his fears, just as earlier in the song he had felt himself to be conquered.

In the first line of 'Madame George', we are 'back on Cyprus Avenue' (caught indeed), 'with a childlike vision leaping into view', and we are in deep semantic ambiguity. The 'childlike vision' is of course Morrison's, but whether it's Morrison as a boy or a generic vision of childhood is not clear.

Here is Madame George, 'marching with a soldier boy behind'. If she is dead, then this is her funeral procession. The soldier boy is apparently 'much older' (so, far from the adult drag queen of standard interpretation, Madame George might be a child) and he's 'drinking wine', which must surely make it difficult to march. Six lines into the song and already we are completely lost on the literal level. And even the identity of the central character alters. Halfway through, 'Madame George' becomes 'Madame Joy', the subject of a related song on Morrison's 1998 compilation of unused material, *The Philosopher's Stone*. Just as mysteriously she then turns back into 'Madame George' and, before the song is out, back into 'Madame Joy' again.

And so it is worth asking whether there is room among the various interpretations for one that places Morrison himself as Madame George. Perhaps he's the child playing dress-up, perhaps he's the soldier boy too, who grows up and drinks wine; perhaps this is his story. His first name, after all, is George. The gentle nostalgia is certainly to do with leave-taking ('get on the train', 'say goodbye'), but it is also about being in the eternal present, the 'now' of memory. So Morrison is simultaneously leaving and coming home. What he is not doing, however, is writing standard autobiography. Rather, he is expressing contradictory states of being, and glimpses of perfection and imperfection based on (presumably, although not even necessarily) real experience. Exaltation is the key — not so much reminiscence as revelation, the Belfast streets leading the 23-year-old man to some Arcadia far away.

Childhood

So at one level, we may regard *Astral Weeks* as the implicit announcement of the start of a musical and emotional journey. Morrison would be twenty years further away from his youth by the time he arrived at his destination in 'reality', singing Irish songs about an Irish childhood ('I'll Tell Me Ma') with an Irish folk band, the Chieftains, on an album called *Irish Heartbeat*. But whether he recognised it or not, this had always been one of his goals. 'I'll Tell Me Ma', like the other (and better) songs on *Irish Heartbeat*, is performed with a winning mixture of Irish innocence and American soul/blues experience, Morrison singing at first rather carefully, then with increasing abandon.

Listening to his voice and technique applied to this, a skipping song that, as a child, he would have heard sung by the girls in his street, one is reminded of the sudden appearance of the children's chorus with its 'Bimm-bamm' bells in Mahler's third symphony. Morrison's music is similarly inclusive. Just because it often deals in first and last things does not mean it must eschew the ordinary or even the infantile. On the contrary, this engagement with everyday and childlike matters underscores and ultimately bolsters the profundity of his work. Often his songs are at their most profound when staring deep into the singer's own youth, because it is from there that he can venture the greatest imaginative distances.

So Van Morrison carries his childhood and adolescence around with him to an unusual degree. Even his legendary taciturnity in the face of an interviewer — or, some nights, an audience — might as well be a prolongation of teenage attitude. More impressionable than most, the pubescent Van was, we imagine, the sort of lad who read and listened to everything, who was inquisitive, insatiable, surly, vulnerable and sometimes a bit pretentious.

The evidence is in the songs he still writes, which at one level are a form of adolescent name-dropping: William Blake and Sidney Bechet, Arthur Rimbaud and the Rosicrucians, Alan Watts and Hank Williams are all visitors to Morrison lyrics. In a single verse of 'Cleaning Windows', Van invokes the names not only of blues greats Leadbelly, Blind Lemon Jefferson, Sonny Terry, Brownie McGhee and Muddy Waters, but also of Christmas Humphreys, the author of *Zen Buddhism*, and Jack Kerouac. Sometimes the tributes come in the form of a straight list, as in 'Max Wall'. This 1989 song, which has never appeared on a commercial release, consists of little more than the names of British comedians that once amused the young Van: 'Harry Worth, Frankie Howerd, Norman Wisdom, Tommy Cooper'; the chorus is 'Max Wall, Max Wall, Max Wall, Max Wall', a reference to one of music hall's saddest clowns. Similarly, on *Enlightenment*, released the following year, the song 'In the Days Before Rock 'n' Roll' mentions all the European stations on Morrison's old transistor radio. If these lists had only contained the names of important figures from literature or the blues, they would certainly have been redolent of Morrison's (well-spent) youth, but might otherwise have been dismissed as mere name-dropping. But that doesn't begin to explain a rollcall that reads: 'Luxembourg, Athlone, Budapest, AFN, Hilversum, Helvetia'. This is not spoken by someone who is out to impress; it's a list that is etched on a memory, the elephantine memory of an obsessive, train-spotting mystic.

Childhood

On 'Got to Go Back', from one of his most unashamedly beautiful records — 1986's *No Guru, No Method, No Teacher* — Morrison sings about his need to return to the past. Although couched in terms of a physical and geographical return, the lyrics, which begin with a description of the view from his classroom window back in Orangefield, describe a sentimental journey back to Morrison's boyhood. He goes home from school and listens to Ray Charles sing 'I Believe to My Soul', then he heads out into 'the street', where the air is still clean (as, presumably, it isn't today). 'Don't play anything sentimental,' Morrison sings without a trace of irony, 'it'll make me cry.' The harmony of 'Got to Go Back' is as static as that of the childhood songs on *Astral Weeks* and nearly all his other childhood songs, and it moves with a gently seductive waltz-like lilt. These songs are generous. Morrison does not want to return alone to the past, he wants to take us with him, and so he becomes a salesman and tour guide for 1950s East Belfast.

The reference to 'the street', for example, is a recurrent image in Morrison's work. It features in nearly all the songs about childhood, either as a specific map reference (such as Cyprus Avenue, the Ballystockart Road, Sandy Row, the Castlereagh Road and Hyndford Street) or as a symbol for happier times. So there he is, standing on the street, or more likely walking down it. Sometimes it's a backstreet, which is often enough wet with rain and occasionally white with snow, and while the street might have a 'dark end', it is generally benign, offering a long-gone sense of community when everyone knew their neighbours and no one ever locked a front door. The street 'knew your name', and times were simpler.

A soul in wonder

Indeed, as Morrison sings on 'It Once Was My Life' from *The Healing Game,* life was complete 'when my message was just the street'. There are dozens of references to streets in these songs and they nearly all signify 'home' — which means the home of Morrison's boyhood.

In addition to the places, specific and general, invoked in the songs, there are also musical references to his formative years in Belfast. Of course these include straight cover versions of songs from his youth — folk songs and blues, jazz standards, cowboy songs and hymns — but even some of the accompaniments to Morrison's own compositions draw on material he would have heard on the radio in the 1950s and early 1960s. The title track of *The Healing Game*, for instance, makes ecstatic use of two phrases from the Ira Gershwin–Vernon Duke standard 'I Can't Get Started', playing them over and over as the song soars to its climax. Another example is *Beautiful Vision*'s 'Dweller on the Threshold', where a trumpet quotes 'The March of the Siamese Children' from Rodgers and Hammerstein's *The King and I*, a 1962 hit for British trumpeter and band leader Kenny Ball. Then on *Down the Road* (2002) and *What's Wrong With This Picture?* (2003), Morrison puts words to tunes by another British jazz man of the same era, Acker Bilk, clarinettist and leader of the Paramount Jazz Band, who guests on the tracks. Born and raised in Somerset in the west of England, Bilk had a hit in 1959 with a song called 'Summer Set'. It is this tune that Morrison sings on *What's Wrong*, and though he calls his version 'Somerset', he is able to make use of Bilk's original pun in his lyric, the memory of a fleeting holiday romance lingering even 'when the summer set'. The same song also carries an affectionate echo of Bilk's biggest hit, the 1961 tune 'Stranger on

Childhood

the Shore', as Morrison's lovers go walking together 'all along the sand'.

There is no obvious reason for these lyrical and musical appropriations and references, particularly for the more fleeting quotes, yet they can only be deliberate. Perhaps they serve no real function at all except to pin down a specific memory, just as his litanies of British comedians and European radio stations evoke certain times, certain places, certain feelings. Of course, were this the case, it would surely be enough. But some of the musical quotations seem to have additional referential purposes. The instrumental hook on 'Got to Go Back', for example, is so strongly reminiscent of 'The Trolley Song' from the musical *Meet Me in St Louis*, particularly the line 'Clang, clang, clang went the trolley', that it's no surprise to learn that Belfast still had trams for much of Van Morrison's childhood.

And the references in his lyrics are often very precise indeed. 'Take me way, way, way back', Morrison says at the beginning of 'On Hyndford Street' (from *Hymns to the Silence*), which is more a poem than a song, and he supplies a list of coordinates for the journey: 'across Beechie River', 'up Cherry Valley from North Road Bridge', 'down by the pylons'. This is a very controlled, gently spoken reminiscence and it draws on familiar images and phrases: we are in 'the days before rock 'n' roll', 'tuning in to Radio Luxembourg' and picking apples from gardens of 'the houses on Cyprus Avenue'. There is a palpable quiet late on summer nights, Morrison tells us, and he asks if we can 'feel' that silence.

'On Hyndford Street' is the centrepiece of this 1991 double album. On the surface, it is perhaps his most overtly religious collection, but the spirituality it exudes is broader than might be suggested by the many apparently Christian references. Morrison's spirituality, like everything else about him, is founded on deep nostalgia. As he speaks, the soft wash of synthetic sound behind his voice has the quality and rather aimless harmonic structure of an organist's extemporisation in a church service or at a revivalist meeting. Morrison, you suddenly realise, is giving his testimony. He is telling us about his personal reality, which is rooted in the past but is 'always now', and as usual he is asking his listeners to go along with him to this paradise on earth that was East Belfast in the 1950s.

This Edenic view of childhood is nowhere more evident than on the title track of Morrison's 1984 album *A Sense of Wonder*. Like all Van's childhood songs since *Astral Weeks*, 'A Sense of Wonder' is long, and there is an epic, questing quality to both the lyrics and the music. We feel we are journeying with the singer (in his 'greatcoat'), and this time the journey takes us back not only to his childhood but to a particular adventure. Childhood brings adventures almost every day, but this one seems special, its significance, as so often with Morrison, mystical. The singer travels 'down' into the past 'though the days of leaves' until he reaches the 'blooming wonder' of youth; but he continues, 'on and on and on', until he reaches the mystical vision for which he has been searching.

This far-reaching quest for the vision, however, means that Morrison's verbal imagery is frequently ambiguous. Sometimes one suspects this is deliberate, but at other times it seems arbitrary and simply the result of a poor choice of words. It is as if Van *feels* his lyrics instead of thinking them through, the resulting verbal imprecision responsible for a good deal of his fans' head-scratching. But Morrison's singing is seldom ambiguous or imprecise. Even when it is impossible to divine the meaning from reading the words on the page (or the CD sleeve), the sound of Morrison's voice generally banishes doubt. When it doesn't convey the meaning, it certainly conveys the spirit.

Each line of the verse begins on C (chord IV), and this lends the song a degree of poignancy, as the music continually reaches for the home key of G. Above this repeating harmonic pattern, Morrison's voice explores the possibilities of the melodic line. He hovers around F#, allowing himself to be lifted up again and again to the G, thus completing the octave with the harmony. Finally, as he repeats the line about describing the leaves, he breaks out of the octave, moving up briefly to A.

'A Sense of Wonder' contains some of Morrison's most rapturous singing on a studio album and some of his most melodically inventive, either in the studio or onstage. Backing him here is the Irish folk-rock band Moving Hearts, and it is hard not to hear this track and the instrumental that follows it — named 'Boffyflow and Spike' after two of the characters he has just sung about — as creative precursors of Morrison's work with the Chieftains. Certainly as Keith Donald's saxophone and Davy Spillane's uillean pipes trade phrases on 'A Sense of Wonder', they seem to inspire greater melodic feats from the singer, an ecstasy of homecoming generated by the lyrics, the repeated harmonic progression and the soaring voice. When the ecstasy finally dies down, Morrison speaks another of his litanies of childhood memorabilia: places and people, characters, both real and celluloid. The reference to Johnny Mack Brown, for example, is to the star of dozens of B-grade cowboy movies, the local cinema being a regular Saturday morning haunt for mid-century working-class children. (Another cowboy, Tom Mix, is among the Beatles' heroes on the cover of *Sgt Pepper*.) Morrison's final list consists of favourite confectionery: 'gravy rings, Wagon Wheels, barmbracks, snowballs . . .'.

The central image, though ultimately perplexing in its meaning, is certainly touching, and not least for the poetic diction Morrison employs to describe 'the leaves'. 'Rich, red browney' and 'half-burnt orange' are specific enough phrases in their evocation of autumn, but why the singer should want to describe the leaves in the first place for 'Samuel and Felicity', and just who Samuel and Felicity are (or, for that matter, Spike and Boffyflow), is anyone's guess. They seem every bit as real as the places Morrison mentions in the first verse — Newtonards and Comber, and the Ballystockart Road — or as the Castle Picture House and Davey's Chipper at the end of the song, but they are as much about *feelings* as they are about reality.

As for the chorus, one must inevitably ask who this 'I' is that comes 'to lift your fiery vision bright' and 'to bring you a sense of wonder in the flame'. And who, for that same matter, is 'you'? In the strictly literal context of the song, 'I' might be the same 'I' who went walking in his greatcoat and described the leaves, and by the same token 'you' (which in any case might be plural) possibly refers to Samuel and Felicity. But there is a different quality to this chorus; there is something

Childhood

frankly Pentecostal both in the imagery and in the repetition of 'didn't I come . . . ?'. As for the 'fiery vision' with 'wonder in the flame', the connection with the colour of the autumnal leaves is clear, but perhaps it's more than that. It is as if Blake's infernal world of experience has been brought into collision with Morrison's childhood innocence and wonder. And in moments like that, one realises the deceptive passion that the songwriter brings to his recollections of the past. They are nostalgic songs, certainly, but every so often, it's as if the memory of them burns into the very soul of the singer.

So ever since *Astral Weeks*, Morrison's songs have been full of his past, as though back in 1968 the young singer was consciously employing musical autobiography as a starting point for spiritual quest. More than two decades later, 'On Hyndford Street' was named after the street on which Morrison himself lived. Sandy Row and the Castlereagh Road, Orangefield School and Davey's Chipper — it's not stretching things too far to suggest that a visitor setting foot for the first time in Belfast would need little more than a good working knowledge of Van Morrison's songs in order to feel at home. It would be like arriving in Dublin with a copy of James Joyce's *Ulysses* tucked under your arm, a book that was actually written in the sunnier climes of continental Europe. For the best guide is often the one who, geographically and chronologically, has moved on, and observed from afar.

MUSICAL HEROES

The image on the front of Van Morrison's 2002 album *Down the Road* features the display window of a small record shop. It is full of old LP covers and the sign reads: 'Memorabilia & Records'.

Down the Road was by no means the first rock album to have a carefully constructed stage-set of a cover. The Beatles' *Sgt Pepper's Lonely Hearts Club Band* is the most obvious example of elaborate cover art designed to reveal background information about the performers, the cut-out heads of Karlheinz Stockhausen, Carl Gustav Jung and W.C. Fields jostling for position amid a sea of other more or less famous faces. These, we are told, were a selection of the Beatles' own heroes, and they ranged from sporting figures to movie stars, from avant-garde composers and psychologist/philosophers to comedians. The cover of *Down the Road* is an equivalent act of homage, but it is subtler, more evocative and more personal than the *Sgt Pepper* montage of thirty-five years before, because the shopfront itself is as important as the 'heroes', the album covers. We find ourselves peering into a reconstruction of a scene from Van Morrison's youth. It is night-time; the illuminated window display invites us in, the light beyond the darkened doorway beckons. We imagine the teenage Van beguiled by a shop such as this. For him it is more than just a record shop, of course. It is a magical place, a private hideaway, a music conservatory, and a shrine. And it offers a key to understanding Morrison's life's work.

Van Morrison became a teenager in the decade that invented teenagers. The very year he reached double figures, Nicholas Ray's film *Rebel Without A Cause* was released and shortly afterwards its star, James Dean, 'took that ride' that killed him; Richard Brooks's film *The Blackboard Jungle* (with 'Rock Around the Clock' over its opening credits) contained a scene in which teenage students smashed their teacher's collection of jazz 78s. That was 1955. The following year, Elia Kazan's *Baby Doll* appeared in cinemas, Little Richard arrived in the pop charts with a song that began 'A wop bop a lu bop a lop bam boom', and Elvis Presley had his first number one with 'Heartbreak Hotel'. *Time* magazine condemned *Baby Doll* as 'possibly the dirtiest American-made motion picture that has ever been legally exhibited', while the *New York Post* quoted Frank Sinatra's opinion that rock music was 'a rancid smelling aphrodisiac . . . martial music of every delinquent on the face of the earth'.

Very likely there has always been a generation gap, but in the 1950s the gap was a chasm. Pop music, in particular, typified the gaping divide. As recently as the 1940s popular music had meant swing bands, and these had appealed to all ages. Music came via radio; families generally had only one of these (the portable transistor was an invention of the '50s), and so within an individual family, everyone tended to listen to the same music. The popularity of the Glenn Miller Orchestra, then, was not a generational matter — by and large, teenagers liked 'In the Mood' as much as their grandparents. By 1955, however, that had all begun to change.

Teenagers suddenly had their own music, and part of its appeal was the fear and loathing it inspired in older generations. The extraordinary explosion of pop music that would come in the '60s was driven by the teenagers of the previous decade, people who had been exposed to the first wave of rock 'n' roll while impressionable adolescents. Van Morrison, highly impressionable, was one of these adolescents, but as always with this artist, there are important differences between his experience and that of most of his contemporaries. For before he ever encountered rock 'n' roll, he'd already been exposed to blues, country-and-western music and jazz via his father's record collection. He sang hymns in church with his mother, and it was probably also his mother who first sang the young Van traditional Irish songs. Important as early rock 'n' roll might have been in forging Morrison's musical personality, the other childhood influences seem to have been more important still.

For the average British teenager, American pop music came via two quite separate routes. It is hard to believe now, given the United States' subsequent world domination in popular culture, but in the mid 1950s, US recordings were hard to find in British shops, and pop music was available on imported vinyl or not at all. Often you had to know someone, and it certainly helped to be living in a sea port — such as

Belfast or Liverpool — that had a steady flow of traffic with the USA. Of course, as the momentum behind rock 'n' roll grew, the records began to arrive and so did the performers (Bill Haley and the Comets playing onstage as the young audience ripped the seats out of the Belfast Empire in 1957). From 1956, however, a discrete, local phenomenon began to bring American folk music into British homes.

Skiffle was a distinctive musical hybrid, roughly three parts American country blues to one part British music hall (with just a dash of country and western). Lonnie Donegan was far and away the most important of these skiffle acts. His early hits were mostly Leadbelly songs such as 'Rock Island Line' and 'Bring a Little Water, Sylvie', given a brisk, slick and, it must be admitted, somewhat sanitised treatment. Donegan would later have hits with the novelty songs 'My Old Man's a Dustman' and 'Does Your Chewing Gum Lose its Flavour on the Bedpost Overnight?', but not until he had inspired the formation of an estimated 50,000 skiffle groups, the length and breadth of the United Kingdom. One of these groups was the Quarrymen, started by John Lennon in Liverpool in 1956 and shortly to feature Paul McCartney and George Harrison.

Morrison has spoken and written about his enthusiasm for skiffle, and in January 2000 he released *The Skiffle Sessions: Live In Belfast 1998*, an album recorded in concert with Lonnie Donegan and Chris Barber. Morrison's relationship to skiffle was ambiguous from the start, for while Donegan was busy introducing the youth of Britain to the blues of Leadbelly, Sonny Terry and Brownie McGhee, the young Ivan Morrison was already well acquainted with this material. Through his father George's record collection, notable for its American imports, Van had gained a detailed knowledge of country blues as well as figures from urban blues and country and western. Lightnin' Hopkins, Jimmie Rodgers and, perhaps above all, Hank Williams were other firm favourites in the Morrison household.

By 1955, Leadbelly, Rodgers and Williams were already dead (Rodgers had been dead for more than two decades), and none of them could ever have been called mainstream, even in their lifetimes — even in the United States. So these were somewhat recherché passions that Van and his father shared. And perhaps that was half the point of it. When Van was five, George, like many Irishmen before him, went to America, intending to find work in the automobile factories of Detroit (the episode is referred to in 'Choppin' Wood' on *Down the Road*). Van was an only child and his father's departure must have been painful. Did George attempt to ease the pain by involving Van in his hopes for a new start? Did he pass on his enthusiasm for all things American (including westerns, both on celluloid and in print) as a way of making his son a partner in this enterprise? Van and his mother waited at home, expecting to be sent for, but the call never came and eventually George returned to Belfast. Did the boy fear that his father would depart again? Was his fascination with the contents of George's record collection an attempt to ensure that they would remain united, at least, in musical esoterica?

Given his exposure to recordings of authentic blues and country music, it seems surprising in some ways that the young Van was as delighted by Lonnie Donegan's ersatz versions as

Musical heroes

he seems to have been. But then the list of musicians that Morrison acknowledges has always constituted a broad church, and the names of his musical heroes do not seem to have altered much over his lifetime. It is tempting to use these heroes, many of whose names are mentioned in Morrison's songs, as a way into understanding his words and music. Morrison's music has always refused categorisation — clearly he is a man who has little time for pigeonholes — but that is not to say his work is devoid of influence. On the contrary, spotting the influences on Morrison is one of those activities that take place whenever two or three of his fans are gathered together. So to what extent is it assisted by the list of musicians mentioned in the songs themselves?

In an attempt to sum up such clues, if clues they are (and a few of them, it must be admitted, quickly prove to be red herrings), one might subdivide the names into various groups. Probably the most significant single group consists of blues musicians, who in addition to the names mentioned above include Big Bill Broonzy, John Lee Hooker, Blind Lemon Jefferson, Muddy Waters and Sonny Boy Williamson. All of them are mentioned in at least one Van Morrison song; Muddy Waters is mentioned in three. There are also the soul and gospel singers: James Brown, Solomon Burke, Gene Chandler, Ray Charles, Sam Cooke, Mahalia Jackson, Wilson Pickett and Jackie Wilson. And the following jazz musicians rate mentions: Louis Armstrong, Chet Baker, Count Basie, Sidney Bechet, Billie Holiday, Jay McShann, Milton 'Mezz' Mezzrow, Jelly Roll Morton, Charlie Parker, Frank Sinatra, Jimmy Witherspoon and Lester Young. Four of the soul singers are named (and quoted) in the coda of 'Real Real Gone'

(*Enlightenment*, 1990), while around half the references to jazz musicians come in just one song, 'The Eternal Kansas City' from 1977's *A Period of Transition*. This tendency to form lists in individual songs demonstrates the unreliability of taking a statistical approach to Morrison's influences, but it doesn't alter the fact that the presence of around thirty namechecks of blues, soul and jazz musicians is unique in the output of one who is ostensibly regarded as a rock musician. Indeed, the presence of the names provides evidence — and this might be half the point of them — that Morrison is more than a rock musician. (A complete inventory of names appears in this book's second appendix, and includes Claude Debussy, Edith Piaf and the Nelson Riddle Orchestra.)

Yet it is not always easy to spot the connection between the citing of a name and the sound of Morrison's music. For example, while it might be true that, in addition to Radio Luxembourg, the young Van also listened to 'Debussy on the Third Programme', as he claims in 'On Hyndford Street', you could waste a lot of time searching his songs for the wholetone scales and symbolist allusions that are synonymous with the French composer.

Some of these names are surely little more than wistful recollections of music that impressed Morrison at some point in his life. But mostly this catalogue of enthusiasms points to specific influences on Morrison's own work, and identifying them goes a long way towards explaining the genetic code behind his hybrid art.

Morrison himself has identified the storytelling quality of Leadbelly's songs as the greatest influence on him, and this seems perfectly appropriate in terms of his early childhood exposure to the material and the connection with his father. Children expect their fathers to provide them with stories. In purely musical terms, however, the blues influence comes not so much from Leadbelly and Sonny Terry, as from the urban, electric blues that developed in Chicago in the 1940s and '50s.

The two most blatant musical debts that Morrison owes to singers are to Muddy Waters and John Lee Hooker, both of whom were born in rural Mississippi during the second decade of the twentieth century, but ended up in Chicago and lived long enough to take the stage with Morrison himself, rather frequently in Hooker's case. John Lee's influence on Morrison's style of singing seems to have been twofold. There is Hooker the blues shouter and there is Hooker the mystic. In Morrison's work, the mystical style of singing is strongly connected to Irish traditional music, but the tougher, terser vocal style is specifically a blues influence, and it is equally informed by the singing of Muddy Waters, who indeed might be said to typify the Chicago sound.

Both Muddy and John Lee affected a kind of urban holler, a staccato blues shout that could be belligerent or sexual, and that, much of the time, was both. You hear it on Muddy Water's 'Hoochie Coochie Man' and 'Mannish Boy': the tone is rasping, individual words are punched, the ends of phrases are abruptly torn off. Morrison has employed this sort of vocal delivery on songs throughout his career, from 'Gloria' in 1967 through to *Down the Road*'s 'Talk Is Cheap', the majority of his albums containing at least one item that can best be understood with reference to the Chicago blues, while some draw heavily on the source.

A soul in wonder

In concert, Morrison is liable to throw in examples of authentic American blues, r&b and soul standards (as opposed to his own songs in those styles), and consequently it is on his live albums that one tends to hear his best blues, r&b and soul singing. On *It's Too Late to Stop Now*, taken from 1973 concerts in Los Angeles and London, and one of the greatest live albums ever released, an ultra-confident Morrison belts out two Sonny Boy Williamson songs, Ray Charles's 'I Believe to My Soul' and Bobby 'Blue' Bland's 'Ain't Nothin' You Can Do', the furious chorus of which is particularly memorable. It is an incendiary performance, and yet much of the pleasure it generates in the listener comes from those moments that are slowly smouldering rather than actually ablaze. Operating at about half the speed of the Rolling Stones' version of the song, Van gives a sultry and supremely controlled rendition of Willie Dixon's 'I Just Want to Make Love to You'. He projects the melodic line in a clipped, almost staccato manner, that emulates his Chicago heroes, but all his energy is focused inwards; he trades phrases with John Platania's guitar, and together they flirt with the audience. Most memorably, he repeatedly takes the performance down to a whisper, going off-mike each time he reaches the song's title and punchline. He is playing at seeming vulnerable, shy of announcing his desire, but he is firmly in control of both the song and the situation it describes. As the teasing reaches its climax (by which time some members of the audience are hesitantly singing along), Morrison sings 'I just want to make —', the blank filled in by a single, gentle 'plunk' from pizzicato strings.

Morrison is at home with this material, and he mixes original songs with these 'standards', moving easily on the record from Sam Cooke's 'Bring it on Home to Me' to his own 'Saint Dominic's Preview' to Sonny Boy Williamson's 'Take Your Hands Out of My Pocket' (although they may well have been recorded on different nights and different sides of the Atlantic). It is equally apparent, however, that, in the company of his backing band, the Caledonia Soul Orchestra, Van is investing much of his own material with a blues/soul sensibility. Of course, songs such as 'Gloria' and *His Band and the Street Choir*'s 'Domino' and 'I've Been Working' are already blues-related, their line structures and chord changes based on identifiable templates. But it is not the performances of these songs, hard-driven and direct as they are, that particularly stand out. The greatest performances on *It's Too Late to Stop Now* are of the slow, introspective songs, and Morrison invests these with an emotional power that seems to be born of the blues. One might speculate, indeed, that the genuine blues material with which he has prefaced the songs has allowed the singer to limber up for the startlingly intense performances of 'Listen to the Lion' and 'Cyprus Avenue'.

'Listen to the Lion' sets out innocently enough in this live recording. The first half of the performance might even be described as playful. 'I shall search my very so-wo-wo-wo-wo-wo-wo-woul', Morrison sings, peppering his delivery with little self-mocking harrumphs. Around two-thirds of the way through the song, there is a brief outburst of roaring. In the original studio performance of this song, on the 1972 album *Saint Dominic's Preview*, this roaring comes to dominate the music, but here in concert Van quickly checks himself. The listener who knows the studio version expects an imminent eruption of noise, but it never comes. The final two minutes simply grow quieter and quieter. The lion, after all, is 'inside of' him, and the intensity of Morrison's performance here tames it until it is still and silent. Morrison is not famous for holding back in performance — at least, not in his more memorable performances — but here it is precisely his restraint that is on show, and it adds immeasurably to the power of his singing.

Restraint was also the hallmark of the other side of John Lee Hooker, the mystic. Particularly later in his life, Hooker became a past master of the interior stream of consciousness, the sad, quiet, slow blues ramble. Van had been doing this sort of thing since *Astral Weeks* in 1968. (After all, what else is 'Beside You'?) It is not impossible, even, that some of the influence here was two-way, when one remembers that Hooker made his own version of Morrison's 'T.B. Sheets'.

Their deeply affecting duet on Hooker's 'I Cover the Waterfront', from his 1991 album *Mr Lucky*, finds the two singers at the top of their form. The tempo is slow; the chord changes are simple, regular, repetitive; there is a static, hypnotised quality to the whole track as Hooker's confidential, closely miked voice vouchsafes a performance of astonishing intimacy. Morrison's contribution is only marginally less introverted, and both singers ornament their vocal lines with a baroque intensity. Booker T. Jones's organ is the other vital contributing factor to this performance, which is pitched somewhere between a dramatic *scena* played out in slow motion and a supplicatory hymn. When Hooker sings, Jones's simple chords are objective, supportive and devoid of vibrato. When Morrison joins in after a couple of minutes, there is a brief touch of vibrato from the organ, adding some further

Musical heroes

colour to the new timbre of Van's voice. Finally, at the climax of the song, describing the much-anticipated arrival of the ship, 'rolling so, so, so slow', and the appearance of the woman 'coming down the gangway', the track achieves its subtle climax. The organ chords climb stepwise into the next octave, in anticipation of Morrison's 'Thank you Lord for bringing my baby back home to me', and then it swells both in volume and tone, the faster, more intense vibrato drawing attention to the very identity of the instrument — suddenly we're in church — and thus emphasising the hymn-like quality of the song.

Blues shares its typical three-chord structure with most Anglo–Celtic folk songs; and, albeit with occasional embellishments, this is also the harmonic blueprint of many hymns. Add to this the fact that all three musical forms depend on relatively simple, strophic (that is, rhythmically repetitious) metres, and a degree of lyrical repetition, and it starts to become clear how Van Morrison can pass from one style to another and occasionally inhabit all three simultaneously.

If an appreciation of blues, soul and jazz came from Morrison's father, it was most likely his mother Violet who was responsible for Van's exposure to traditional music and hymns. Perhaps the instilment began earlier, because the influence of Irish folk song and Protestant hymnody seems to lie deeper in Morrison's musical unconscious. He might have recorded only two genuine hymns ('Be Thou My Vision' and 'Just a Closer Walk with Thee', in 1991), as opposed to an entire album of traditional folk songs, but his tendency to compose songs in a hymn-like form has been evident for a long time.

The hymns feature, appropriately, on the *Hymns to the Silence* double album, but elsewhere there are veiled and quite probably subconscious references to other hymns. One example, twenty years before 'Be Thou My Vision', is on that most gentle of all Morrison's love songs, 'Tupelo Honey'. That track's recurring flute riff is virtually identical to the opening line of Hubert Parry's melody ('Repton') for the hymn 'Dear Lord and Father of Mankind' by John G. Whittier, a popular selection from the Protestant hymnal, *Songs of Praise*. Given Morrison's willingness to quote single lines from the popular songs of his youth (Kenny Ball's hit 'The March of the Siamese Children' et al), it seems reasonable to believe that this is also a deliberate reference. The quotation may be as meaningless as one imagines that Kenny Ball quote to be, but it is also now possible to read 'Tupelo Honey' as a song of praise, if only to Van's wife Janet Planet ('she's an angel').

It might be relevant that Parry (1848–1918) also composed the familiar music to William Blake's 'Jerusalem', frequently sung in Britain as a Protestant hymn. In spite of its association with the outmoded chauvinism of the Last Night of the Proms, this song is in effect a socialist anthem — Blake's words about 'dark satanic mills' having been penned at the start of the industrial revolution, while it was first sung in Parry's setting at a 1916 suffragette rally. 'And was Jerusalem builded here?' asks Blake. The answer, obviously, is no; but the intention nevertheless is to build it 'in England's green and pleasant land'. Morrison quotes the tune at the end of 'A Town Called Paradise', on 1986's *No Guru, No Method, No Teacher*, and his band often interpolates the melody in live performances of

'Summertime in England' (from *Common One*, 1980), a song that itself asks the question, 'Did you ever hear about Jesus walkin' down by Avalon?'

On *Down the Road*, 'The Beauty of the Days Gone By' is a more obvious example of a hymn-like song. Not only does it exhibit a pronouncedly strophic form, relatively formal syntax and some specific allusions to the diction of hymnody ('because my cup doth overflow'), but there is also a direct parallel to a hymn by Isaac Watts. 'When I Survey the Wondrous Cross' is one of the most famous of all Protestant hymns — Charles Wesley once maintained he would have given all of his own hymns to have written it — and it is inconceivable that Van would not know it and have sung it as a child. Both its metre and its opening line structure are the same as in Morrison's song: 'When I survey the wondrous Cross' / 'When I recall just how it felt / When I went walking down by the lake'. At the same time, the 6/8 lilt of the melody evokes folk song (as does Edward Miller's melody, 'Rockingham', most commonly sung to Watts's hymn), and Morrison's delivery of the vocals, with its clipped phrase endings, only adds to that lilt — you could actually waltz to it — taking the music simultaneously in another direction.

But that is what one often finds with Van Morrison's music. The influences that inform his songs tend to be tangled and hard to separate. This is particularly true when the influences are hymns and folk songs. Neither of these musical forms is ever referred to in the specific name-checking manner that jazz, soul and blues musicians are celebrated, and perhaps the reason for this is that both folk song and hymnody are fundamental to Morrison, taken in, as it were, with his mother's milk. In consequence he is himself broadly unaware of their influence. It is a different matter with blues, jazz, soul, gospel, country and rock 'n' roll. Each of these American styles of music involved a degree of discovery, if only following the placing of a stylus in a record groove, and it might be just such moments of epiphany that Morrison continues to celebrate with his name-checks.

To a great extent, this is a matter of Van being an enthusiast. To his boot straps, he's one of those people who is not happy until *you* like a particular song as much as *he* does. At one level, this is a form of cultural imperialism, but it is also an act of generosity: *You don't know Sonny Boy Williamson? Amazing. Okay, I'll sing you one of his songs . . . You liked that? Good. You want to know more about the blues? Well, here are the names of some singers you should listen to . . .* If Van Morrison could, he'd make you a compilation tape. Since he can't, he puts those tapes into his songs.

It is the paying of dues, then. It is boundless enthusiasm (cultural imperialism). It is a matter of respect. And here blues, soul and jazz rub right up against the other part of Morrison's childhood. Not just the folk music and the hymns, but the background to the hymns: the Protestant upbringing which, in Northern Ireland, was always proud, always vulnerable, always ready to defend itself, always tempted to pick a fight — like Van Morrison himself, come to think of it. And also the Jehovah's Witnesses, with whom Violet Morrison at least briefly threw in her lot. All that testifying, knocking on doors and trying to interest complete strangers in a copy of *The Watchtower.* (*Good morning, have you heard of Ray Charles? Have you considered letting Sam Cooke into your heart?*)

Musical heroes

By name-checking his heroes, Morrison is also attempting to make converts. But ultimately, of course, the references are not really for us; they are for him. And sometimes they sound like a slightly nervous child saying his prayers. He wants to do the right thing. He doesn't want to leave anyone out. He concentrates hard. Here goes . . . *God bless Mummy and Daddy and Uncle Jim and Auntie Joan and the man up the road and Muddy Waters and John Lee Hooker and Edith Piaf and . . . [yawn] . . . Claude Debussy and . . .*

TRANSCENDENCE AND RELIGION

The best-known live version of one of Morrison's greatest songs, 'In the Garden' (on 1994's *A Night in San Francisco*), sets off at an almost frantic pace. Van's delivery is perfunctory and has a kind of let's-get-it-over-with feel. There's no sense of milking the song for emotion; on the contrary, it's as though the singer is deliberately trivialising the beauty of one of his most moving tunes, tossing it off as if it were just some trifle from the back catalogue. But then, progressively, the band and Van himself seem to become more engaged, the vocals start to distort through cupped hands, a piano solo lifts the mood, and the reeds sing over the top as the song winds its way down into whispered, almost indecipherable vocals, fading into obscurity, then back again to clarity, like the moments before sleep.

Five minutes in, the dream-world of the song has opened out. With only the light, quick rhythm section and fragments

Transcendence and religion

from the other instruments remaining, there are limitless horizons, with the medley format, so common a feature of Morrison's concerts, taking hold. First, we enter 'Allegheny' and look around, finding the spirit (and the name-check) of Sam Cooke in there somewhere. Then Van calls for the distinctly real Brian Kennedy, his regular backing vocalist at the time, to come back on stage and we enter the next musical world, of Sam Cooke's 'You Send Me', a parallel universe, the music still muffled and indistinct, then suddenly clear again. And then, without warning, we snap out of it with Van's incantation of the line 'No guru, no method, no teacher' and a return to the original song. With the band progressively returning from its reverie, 'In the Garden' then moves towards the daylight, in triumph, into the here and now. With all the performers finally focused on the refrain, the pop song has returned from an enchanted world and the concert is brought to a rousing climax as the star heads for the wings and the MC demands applause.

It's through the patient search for these transcendent moments — when spiritual ecstasy and commercial appeal merge into one seamless whole — that Van Morrison's fans endure endless hours of grudging performances and boorish behaviour. And when they happen, there is no one in popular music who can match him, and nothing that can explain how such intensity can emerge from so little apparent intent.

In these moments, Morrison would appear to become the cipher for something higher, the medium through which the message travels. He is like a biblical hero, whose character and background are patently unsuited to the job, but through whose unreliable offices the task must be performed anyway.

A soul in wonder

And in bringing it off consistently over forty years, he seems to offer proof that there is a higher power at work. But what exactly is that higher power? Van himself asks the question continually. Is it God or is it nature? The answer depends on which phase of his career — indeed which album or even individual song — one refers to. Morrison is a pantheist, a pagan, a nature-worshipper, a Christian, a Scientologist, a Jehovah's Witness, a Zen Buddhist, depending on which voice he employs.

Among his peers, only Bob Dylan can compete with Morrison in terms of spiritual — or more particularly, religious — doubt and conviction. God and Van Morrison have been acquaintances over many albums, but on each occasion, they wear different disguises, challenging each other to commit and testify. This spiritual shadow-boxing has sometimes been a source of amusement for his fans, but for Morrison himself, it's another source of torment. Brought up Protestant in sectarian Belfast by a mother who was a sometime Jehovah's Witness, Van tries to believe but ends up asking when he will 'ever learn to live in God'.

Of course these traces of organised religion, these lyrical and musical references to assorted spiritual paths, are no different from the hymn-like tunes and the occasional appearance of gospel choirs. They are 'intertextual' clues from which Morrison's listeners construct the meanings of the songs. With his preacher-like rantings and explicit calls for gods and gurus (or sometimes no gods and no gurus), he establishes his musical foundations in a Christian tradition, before taking it out into the great unknown via the doors of jazz, folk, soul and rock. The point of departure is always manifest, the object — a higher meaning — never in doubt, but how to recognise that point of destination and how to live in it represent the eternal dilemma.

While the wonders of nature and devotion to a Christian god fight for supremacy, Morrison himself searches for the space in which time no longer matters, where silence and eternity reign in a world of perpetual wonder. The means to this end are often the narration of incidents from childhood. It's that moment of hypnotic stasis that we hear in 'On Hyndford Street', from 1991's *Hymns to the Silence*. It's the journey towards silence that characterises the middle section of 'In the Garden'. It's the point of spiritual ecstasy that 'So Quiet in Here' (from 1990's *Enlightenment*) almost, but never quite, achieves.

When it works, time seems to stand still. We might be in a Zen monastery; we might be at Ronnie Scott's club in London at three in the morning; we might be 'caught', stock-still on East Belfast's Cyprus Avenue. Whatever narrative took us there, when we reach that space, a sense of timelessness takes over. It's the point where the curmudgeonly old stager loses himself in his art. But as that live version of 'In the Garden' demonstrates, with the commercial imperative at work, we do not rest there for long before the return to format is activated and the song is brought home.

Always central to such moments is Morrison's voice. For example, in 'Madame George' on *Astral Weeks*, the moment of transcendence also maintains a strong sense of forward propulsion, as the acoustic guitar mechanically strums away at the same three chords. Around this constant, musicians wander lost and bewildered. The flute and violin play flourishes — far too many notes and far too elaborate to indicate anything but mild panic. The stand-up bass follows the general chord pattern, loosely, an outsider looking in on a world he's never encountered before. But over them all, Morrison's voice, snarling and hypnotic, delivers a mantra, the lyrics disintegrating into the now famous 'To love to loves to love to loves' incantation. Rambling, nonsensical, self-important and stylistically chaotic, the song is nevertheless a triumph, because the ear is drawn irresistibly to the grain of Morrison's vocal. It's not a kind voice. The compelling voices rarely are. The political orator commands attention in strident tones. The Southern preacher rants about his vision of God's beauty. Even at its most restrained, Van's voice howls with rage and indignation. It's not a lovely sound, but it is thrilling.

Still, Morrison tries to be humble. In the title track of *Enlightenment* we discover a Zen Van chopping wood while contemplating the sound of one hand clapping. The lyrics, for once, are perfectly transparent, but the heart of the song is that grumbling, folksy vocal emerging with clarity from the new-age keyboard-choir at the opening. So while the words tell us that the singer doesn't know the meaning of the word 'enlightenment', the sound of his voice contradicts the message. It's like some spiritual guide suddenly appearing in the mist, clearly pointing the way.

And yet this is the ultimate paradox in any consideration of spirituality in Morrison's songs. Because what is this guide — this voice — pointing at? Throughout his career, and particularly since the early 1980s, the singer's spiritual quest has regularly touched on Christian religions and sects. In the late 1970s he was celebrating the revivalist fervour in the Kingdom Hall. In the mid 1980s he seems to have had a brief flirtation with L. Ron Hubbard and the Scientologists. A few years later, on 1989's *Avalon Sunset*, he was 'born again' and rapturously singing the praises of God's shining light with that purveyor of all things bright and botox, Sir Cliff Richard. Their collaboration, 'Whenever God Shines His Light', is a poppy little number, but the lyrics are pure hymnal. The believer trusts that 'in the darkest night' and 'in great despair' and 'deep confusion', when he reaches out for God, 'He'll be there'. But rather than just a simple song of praise, the improbable duet goes further, for this God's blessing takes the form of healing 'the sick and . . . the lame'. Speaking in tongues is just around the corner.

Were it not for intervening albums featuring paganism and nature-worship, one would almost suspect from these examples that Van was essentially a man of the flock whose albums should be filed under 'Christian rock'. It's an impression confirmed in *Hymns to the Silence*, which, without being overtly 'sacred' in intent, nevertheless encapsulates so many of Morrison's religious and mystical preoccupations.

Sitting cheek by jowl with tirades against 'professional jealousy', 'parasites', 'hypocrites' and 'people who drain' ('Professional Jealousy', 'Why Must I Always Explain?'), Morrison sings in 'By His Grace' that you have to 'live your religion' through 'trying for the Kingdom on high'. That ultimate state of grace comes 'one day at a time', from somewhere deep inside, when your heart is opened to the Wisdom. Like several other tracks on *Hymns to the Silence*, 'By His Grace' is musically unexceptional, but in its lyrics we hear the same message we have 'time and time again' — that throughout his work there is a consistent, even considered, pattern of religious observance and sentiment that derives directly, although not literally, from the mainstream church liturgies. And yet for all these obvious recurrences of Christian language, imagery and themes throughout a long career, any attempt to align Van himself with Christianity in any one specific form is problematic.

Bob Dylan went through an artistically dubious Christian phase making genuine efforts to practise his new-found beliefs. U2 began their career as an identifiably Christian band, promulgating moral righteousness with military intensity until the religious zeal was superseded temporarily by a fascination with the loneliness of American hotel rooms. But with Van, there is often a sense that the Christianity and the obsession with God is superficial — a tangential relationship, the ultimate name-check. Morrison is at pains to stress that his religious faith can't be summarised by one label or by an adherence to any identifiable faith. It's one of those topics that riles him into demanding, 'Why must I always explain?' Perhaps the best way to describe him — as he himself repeats more than a dozen times in the title track of 1983's *Inarticulate Speech of the Heart* — is as 'a soul in wonder'. But what sort of soul is he? And what sort of wonder does he experience? If Morrison is not, and probably never has been, a conventional, 'practising Christian', how can one explain the overt 'Christianity' of so much of his music, particularly that from the late 1980s and early 1990s?

In interviews, Morrison has said that he was never really concerned about religion when he was growing up, and that he only first became aware of it when he was beaten up one day walking home from school. With typical disinterest he reports that he didn't even know if he was being beaten up for being Protestant or Catholic but that whoever was doing it hated him for being the other. But he knew he was Protestant, of course. East Belfast might have been less sectarian than some other parts of the city, but no one growing up in Belfast in the 1950s could be unaware of the dominating, life-and-death struggle for religious and political dominance that had shaped nearly three centuries of the city's history, and which, within a decade, would escalate to reach new levels of brutality.

What Van does admit is that he went to some of the JW meetings with his mother, and 'Kingdom Hall' (from *Wavelength*, 1978) is a blatant celebration of the separatist, revivalist culture that he encountered there with Violet. The song, which announced Morrison's 'comeback' after just one, disappointing album in the four years prior to it (1977's *A Period of Transition*), begins with a welcome — 'So glad to see you, so glad you're here' — and then an invitation to 'clear inhibition away' and dance 'like we've never been dancing before'. Before you know it, the congregation is 'swinging', 'ringing' and 'singing'. Morrison's version of the Kingdom Hall sounds like the hippest joint in town, well worth all those hours spent traipsing the streets and having front doors slammed in your face. Before long they're really 'shaking it out on the floor' to the strains of 'good rocking music'. If this is autobiography, then it sounds like Elvis Presley and his fellow Southern Baptists had some stiff competition from those party-loving Latter Day Saints in 1950s Belfast.

A soul in wonder

Violet Morrison was not always a Jehovah's Witness — it seems to have been a passing phase. But despite her son describing her in 1997 as 'a free-thinker' who wouldn't like being described as 'religious', there is no doubt that she was a practising Christian at certain times in her life, and given that the young Ivan was an only child, and apparently quite a spoilt one, it hardly seems possible that Morrison had anything other than a traditional, perhaps even quite fundamentalist Christian upbringing. But that is not to say he routinely went to church or undertook confirmation. Rather, just as the young Morrison absorbed the language of the King James Bible and the Prayerbook, together with the hymn tunes that influence him still, so he grew up with the social structures and patterns of ritual that Protestantism brings. The issue of whether or not he was a 'practising Christian' is irrelevant. What is relevant is that Morrison imbibed the culture of Protestantism in the house where he grew up. It was, as he himself described his childhood, 'a very churchy atmosphere in the sense that that's the way it is in Northern Ireland'. And for all the apparent haphazardness of his formal worship, the young Van Morrison was engaged in a highly structured, highly disciplined culture of religious observance and ritual.

When Van sings 'Be Thou My Vision' (another *Hymns to the Silence* track), he does so with a sense of determination, soldiering on through the hymn like a dutiful parishioner. And yet the tune itself, originally known as 'Slane' after a hill in County Meath, is a gorgeous thing whose origins (as Paddy Moloney's uillean pipes remind us) date back to eighth-century Ireland. And, one suspects, when Morrison sings the lines 'Be thou my breastplate, my sword for the fight / Be thou my armour and be thou my might', he too might be delving deep into the archaic rituals of Protestantism on which so many of his lyrics and his attitudes are founded. These stentorian incantations for protection (called Lorica in the Irish tradition) could equally apply to the bad-mouthing songs too, which feature with equal prominence on *Hymns to the Silence*.

We might think of Christian ritual as being the exclusive preserve of Catholicism, with its grand ceremonies, symbolic communions, actual confessions and enforced celibacy, not to mention its apocalyptic concepts of hellfire and guilt. But while Protestantism lacks the theatre, in many ways it possesses a far greater sense of codified behaviour. The work ethic that drives Protestantism, at its core, is an almost fanatical application of discipline and ritual. And this is not the preserve of Sunday morning observances but rather an integral part of daily life, twenty-four hours a day, seven days a week. It can take the form of music practice for ecclesiastical or community performance, or doing good deeds, or attendance at the various services, dotted through the week at appointed times (five per week for Jehovah's Witnesses).

The young Protestant musician knows that one never misses a rehearsal. It's this discipline, this zeal to perform one's duty, that sustains the work ethic, and to this day it sustains Morrison's art. But amid all this duty, there comes a pay-off. Crucially, as every Protestant knows, the very act of participation can prompt a moment of enlightenment — endurance can lead to revelation. It is precisely what occurs in those transcendent moments that happen along, from time to time, in Morrison's music.

A soul in wonder

So, on the one hand, Morrison is a journeyman musician, writing songs because it's how he makes his living, churning them out whether or not he feels inspired (clearly, he often doesn't). On the other hand, he is a mystical poet capable of moments of sublime meditative beauty. And that link between the banal observance of ritual — the concert starts at 8 pm no matter what, and Van must sing for a minimum of seventy minutes — and the occasional moment of transcendence occurs because Morrison is, if only at the level of memory and routine, a Protestant.

In 'Cleaning Windows', one of the most enduring tracks from *Beautiful Vision*, Van declares himself to be 'a working man in my prime', and this is equally true whether he's a window cleaner going 'straight back to work' or a fifteen-year-old playing in a show band in Europe for eight hours a night. As he describes it in 'Why Must I Always Explain?', he gets 'out on the highway and on with the show' because 'it's just a job, you know'. Through that work, God will appear — at least sometimes — but Van will keep pushing whether He appears or not. That's the Protestant work ethic. Ritual leads to religion, not the other way around. Practice becomes prayer. That's the Protestant way. (Catholics do it in reverse.)

NATURE AND LITERATURE

It would be fair to describe Morrison as a 'spiritual' artist, not because his songs argue that humankind is inherently religious, nor because he actively professes a particular faith, but because throughout his work there is always a concept of the existence of a supreme power. This mysterious higher force is always present in his music, but the church is not the place where the revelation is made. In the garden, misty, 'wet with rain' (*No Guru No Method No Teacher*) Morrison feels the presence of Christ in his heart. On Cyprus Avenue (*Astral Weeks*), when time stands still, he is confronted with a 'childlike vision' of infinite wonder. And always, the 'presence' emerges in quiet places.

According to historian Thomas Carlyle, 'Worship is transcendent wonder', and for Morrison that 'sense of wonder' derives from Protestant teaching but is revealed in the landscape. It is there, in the Castlereagh Hills, on a journey to Coney Island, or in those ubiquitous cool, clear crystal waters, that the consciousness rises to the presence of

God. As the American philosopher and Quaker historian Rufus Matthew Jones put it, at this moment of transcendence, the tangible communion with the Almighty 'floods the soul with joy and bathes the whole inward spirit with refreshing streams of life'. These moments are not typical of all of Van Morrison's work, least of all the soul and r&b tracks, but are encountered particularly on the more 'Celtic' albums such as *Veedon Fleece* (1974), *Common One* (1980), *No Guru, No Method, No Teacher* (1986) and *Hymns to the Silence* (1991). They identify Morrison as a modern-day Protestant preacher, a missionary without a pulpit, possessed of an inherently religious sensibility devoid of the customary outward signs. If he has a guru, a method or a teacher, they are to be found in nature itself.

From certain vantage points in East Belfast the Castlereagh Hills loom large, seemingly a stone's throw away, and they provide a stunning contrast with the urban commercial reality of daily life. Morrison refers to these specific rolling hills in the blatantly autobiographical song 'On Hyndford Street', from *Hymns to the Silence*, but the metaphor pervades his work in general. Even in the middle of a blues number or some big-band soul, there is usually a distant forest or stream or some other natural phenomenon waiting to offer up its healing power to the searcher.

In so many of his songs, we encounter Van standing stock-still in the midst of life, staring up at that mystical place where nature reigns supreme and the world is prelapsarian — simple, pure and restorative. But while the impetus for the recurrent motif is undoubtedly personal, there is a literary heritage underlying it too. It is the world of the Romantic poets who, amidst the technological tyranny of the industrial revolution, of William Blake's 'dark satanic mills', sought for this idyllic place of peace and harmony.

To Morrison, the appeal of William Wordsworth's poem 'The Prelude' in particular, and the work of the Lake Poets more generally, is obvious. The reference appears in arguably his most embarrassing lyric, from *Common One*'s 'Summertime in England' — 'Did you ever hear about Wordsworth and Coleridge, baby? / They were smokin' up in Kendal', he sings, referring to the Lake District town. Yet there is little doubt that for Morrison the emotions generated by the experience of nature are the same as those evoked more than 150 years earlier by the Romantics. Wordsworth and Samuel Taylor Coleridge fled industrialisation to find mystical renewal in the direct experience of the wind and the rain. The young Morrison fled the grim, grey shipyards in which his father worked and where, even after he'd recorded with Bert Berns, he might well have ended up himself. He also fled the artificial and mechanical world of rock music to pursue his own quest for some deeper spiritual experience.

Industry and nature, hard work and renewal of the spirit, the mundane and the sublime — all the contradictory obsessions of Morrison's art — come together in the Romantic ethos of the pilgrim wandering through the landscape, filled up inside with a sense of wonder at nature's beauty. And in Morrison's work, it's always an idealised natural world. There's never a polluted stream, there are no power lines obscuring the view, no super-highways cutting across the meadows. This faultless, nurturing nature, like Morrison's youth, exists in a mythical 'present' and it has a capacity, undiminished by the presence of human beings, to heal and invigorate the senses and the spirit. Nature, indeed, is where the misanthropic Morrison always retreats when 'professional jealousy' and 'big-time operators' and 'people who drain' get the better of him. Because in his landscape there is no human presence at all, just a sense of everlasting life, rain to be cleansed in and fish to be caught.

The landscapes are both specific and universal. Aside from the topographical features of Northern Ireland, Van finds inspiration in American nature too, from the snow in San Anselmo to the honey from the Tupelo gum tree. But nothing compares to the inspiration he gets from the landscape that Wordsworth and Coleridge knew in England. 'Summertime in England' — a sprawling, imperfect monster of a track — is Morrison's quintessential nature song. Here in the countryside where he had made his home, and over a not always appropriate rhythm-and-blues groove, Morrison plants himself firmly in the English pastoral tradition, not just that of the Lake Poets and of Matthew Arnold's poem 'The Scholar Gipsy', but of composers Edward Elgar and Ralph Vaughan Williams and all the other champions of the 'green and pleasant land'. It is here, in this place, as he waits to meet his 'red-robed common one' — common but also 'illuminated' — that thoughts of Jesus prowling the English countryside begin to emerge through the filter of William Blake. Glastonbury, or in Morrison's lexicon 'Avalon', becomes a holy site, his lyrics tapping into the English folk tradition that identified the region as the base for either Jesus' or his disciple Joseph of Arimathea's rumoured English ministry.

And across this sublime landscape, where, as usual, the destination is silence, comes a passing parade of random

Nature and literature

thoughts, about Wordsworth and Coleridge of course ('Summertime in England' is surely Morrison's own 'Prelude'), but also gospel singer Mahalia Jackson and T.S. Eliot. They are not in the landscape, but the landscape evokes in the singer's mind a sense of their historical significance. They are clouds drifting across his mental horizon, not thoughts as such but distant memories, evocative names generating moods and feelings that can't adequately be captured in anything but music. It's easy to lampoon these particular name-checks, but the references to Eliot and Jackson are no more than the cloud that looks like a bear, or an elephant, or a face, and which soon will be blown on by the prevailing breeze. That's when the silence enters, and the breath goes in and out, in and out, in meditation.

For Morrison, nature is the place where time stands still, where, once 'the red-robed common one' and the poets and gospel singers and the flotsam of mental activity have been silenced at last, the eternal can be captured and contemplated in a single mystical moment. It is the world beyond, the Eden or the Avalon of the heart, the garden of paradise that renders misanthropy unnecessary and engenders peace and enlightenment. And when it's so quiet in there, it's easy to recognise the paradox of a man, identified with the loudest art form ever invented, devoting his career to seeking out such moments of tomb-like silence.

For Morrison, this urge towards reconciliation with nature has been a constant feature of his work since *Astral Weeks* in 1968. From the first tracks of that first album, Morrison's characters venture out in falling rain, breathing in and out as high-flying clouds surround them in ecstasy. They drink the cool, clear crystal waters in gardens all wet with rain and from the hillside mountain glide they are laid down in silence, being born again in another time and place and going up to heaven. Decades on, the same motifs emerge, not just in the explicitly mystical albums but even in commercial ventures such as 1989's *Avalon Sunset*. There is some justification then in Morrison's complaint that he tells people the same thing over and over again. In terms of nature, it's perfectly true.

Crucial to Morrison's nature-worship is the role of the seasons. Barely an album passes without references to the time of year, while phrases such as 'golden autumn day' recur frequently, the singer often finding himself knee-deep in fallen leaves. It is rather reminiscent of those age-old traditions in which the seasons were metaphors for the annual patterns of decline and renewal. While he doesn't specifically refer to harvest songs, mummers' plays or May Day celebrations, there seems little doubt that Morrison's Anglo–Celtic art is tapping into this rich vein of cultural history. It is in the modern-day reworking of the pastoral tradition that the folk roots of Morrison's songs are most apparent. It's the world of 'Down by the Salley Gardens' and 'Carrickfergus', where the action happens out of doors, in a garden or by a stream or some other natural phenomenon whose mythic significance reverberates in our lives.

Individual months also bring with them the kinds of natural phenomena that reflect personal moods and emotions. In the title track of 1984's *A Sense of Wonder*, for instance, we hear that 'It's easy to describe the leaves in the Autumn / And it's oh so easy in the Spring / But down through January and February it's a very different thing.' In fact those midwinter months are always a trial in Morrison's music, and never more so than in 'Fire in the Belly' from *The Healing Game* (1997), where the lines 'Gotta get through January / Gotta get through February' become a grim mantra.

The end point is always renewal following those depressing months of January and February, but while the gist is that of rebirth ('To be born again / In another time, in another place' as it is expressed in 'Astral Weeks'), the specific metaphor that is most often employed is that of healing. Morrison's concerts have often ended with the question 'Did you get healed?', and it's the implicit message of songs from all periods of his career, as well as the title of a song from 1987's *Poetic Champions Compose*. The word 'healing' keeps cropping up, and the healing capacity of music was the topic of a forum that Morrison sponsored in 1987. Music heals and nature heals too. They are the two things that touch the 'very soul'.

But it's not just Van's lyrics that evoke nature. There is a sonic quality to many of his songs that creates and re-creates a sense of the natural world. Even in a song such as 'Why Must I Always Explain?', which is one of his most griping numbers (from *Hymns to the Silence*, an album not short of griping sentiments), the music manages to speak of the outdoors because of the presence of uillean pipes. This distinctive sonority seems to embody the spirit of the wind in the face high on the mountain, and even when the pipes themselves are not physically present, Morrison's drifting Celtic soundscapes often leave room for the memory of that sound.

More fundamental is Morrison's own voice — the *Ur*-sonority of his work, to which any study of the songs must continually return. In gruff mode, this voice speaks of the outdoors man, up there doing his 'jig among the rolling hills', to quote from a song on 1979's *Into the Music*. At such moments, he is the folk singer whose phrasing is as spontaneous and untutored as that of the County Derry shepherd boy herding his flock. This particular quality to Morrison's work reaches its apogee on *Irish Heartbeat*, the 1988 collaboration with the Chieftains that must rank as one of the folk tradition's finest modern renewals. Here, singing other people's (indeed, mostly *the* people's) material, Morrison touches the source of so many of his own lyrical and melodic ideas. He's at the country fair, he's on Raglan Road (on yet another autumn day), and he's looking for a boatman to cross the river to where his love lies waiting. At the best of times, Van Morrison is a singer who is always going someplace, always walking somewhere, always cast out into the elements and finding rejuvenation of the spirit there. On *Irish Heartbeat* he is doing all this among his 'own ones'.

An identification with nature is, of course, hardly new in Celtic art. W.B. Yeats and John Millington Synge both found the wilds of Ireland to be metaphors for the human condition. Irish art has achieved many of its finest moments in the shebeen, with the sea pounding away outside, threatening to destroy the humanity sheltering within. Nature is untameable in the greatest Irish art but its life-threatening quality is transformed in Morrison's songs into a gentler, healing capability. While storms might threaten, they are never severe. The wind will blow cold, but the golden day is only one dark night away. Frankly, this is a sentimental view of nature, idealised, sanitised, purged of all danger and transformed into a reassuring fairytale. The rain is a comforter, the wind sweeps away troubles, and if you pull your greatcoat up around your ears you should end up surviving those nasty months of January and February. To the soul in wonder, nature is its own church, the wind and the rain its ministers, and their teachings are of healing and comfort.

In fact the mythological and literary sources of Morrison's natural world are not Irish at all. The myths are English — Arthurian ('knights in armour bent on chivalry', as he observes on the title track of 1971's *Tupelo Honey*) and pre-Arthurian — and so is the literature that describes Avalon (or Glastonbury), Stonehenge and other ancient ruins dimly picked out through the fog of time. These are Morrison's 'haunts of ancient peace'. And in the song that bares this title (on *Common One*), many of the singer's thematic preoccupations merge. The track begins with an undefined, timeless instrumental background, Mark Isham's distant trumpet drifting over some ethereal, spacious bass line that comes as if from distant memory. As the singer enters he is walking, dreaming about ancient times, peace, and the search for love and light. In this meditative space, there is no need for speech, the wind is blowing and the Sunday bells are chiming around the countryside and towns. When we reach the third verse, time travel has seized control of the narrative. Look to your left in this transcendental moment and you'll encounter the Arthurian Holy Grail and, over on your right, is Blake's New Jerusalem.

This return to mystical, idyllic roots characterises so much of Morrison's music and takes so many different forms. Personally, it is the return to his childhood state of wonder in East Belfast. Musically, it is the recollection of all his boyhood r&b idols. Lyrically, it is the invocations of Blake and Yeats and (less directly) Patrick Kavanagh. Historically, it is an imaginative recreation of pre-industrial Britain, with its epic quests in search of redemption. Spiritually, it is a return to the direct experience of God, independent of the mediation of the church, achieved by working dutifully and hard. And geographically, it is the celebration of the natural world, that rolling countryside before the train lines and roads cut their scars across the landscape. This natural environment is Blake's vision of innocence (which is not unlike J. R. R. Tolkien's Shire), where enlightenment is found in simple living and in the blessed relief of the wind and the rain. (Blake's vision of experience comes in a song such as *Hymns to the Silence*'s 'Professional Jealousy'.)

At one level, of course, this is all risible. Here is a working man from Belfast, born within days of the dropping of the atom bombs on Hiroshima and Nagasaki, living through the Cold War and the Irish 'Troubles', and cobbling together a philosophy of life from assorted ancient myths and religions, the whole of it wrapped in obvious clichés. But perhaps this is where Morrison's notorious disinterest and grumpiness play their most important role. When delivered with his distinctive ill-humour, even those songs that, on the page, seem like a rag-bag of anachronisms and warmed-over sentiment are far harder to dismiss. On the contrary, that gruff, unbeautiful voice transforms the material.

Morrison is not the first modern artist who has sought his inspiration in the events and ideas of the distant past. Again the parallel with Ralph Vaughan Williams may not be inappropriate. Amid the ravages of economic depression and world wars, the English composer found a convincing spiritual and aesthetic strength in the musical structures — and even the moral universe — of a long-gone Tudor England and of the English 'folk' themselves. The folk singer is a curious artist. In a sense trapped in time (that is, trapped by tradition), the singer's role is nevertheless one of renewal in the moment. The sentiment of a song might remain the same as it passes through the oral tradition; the notes and the words do not. In that sense, then, Morrison's music inhabits the same cultural space as those mid-twentieth-century English composers who took folk song and the music of the countryside as their point of departure. Both Benjamin Britten and Van Morrison have presented 'Down by the Salley Gardens' after their own fashions. More significant though is the way in which for composers such as Vaughan Williams, Gustav Holst and Britten, working with traditional music affected their own styles. It has been exactly the same for Morrison. In paying obsessive homage to his predecessors, he has succeeded in creating a new sort of song, hybridised, but authentic for all that, and it is the perfect musical vessel for his very personal vision of the world.

In Morrison's world, the sins of humanity are washed away in a superficially banal but philosophically profound sensual communion between the psyche and the hedgerow. In part, of course, this comes from Blake, but any text that champions the cause of the 'natural' past and decries the technological innovations of the present is grist for Morrison's mill.

Kenneth Grahame's children's novel *The Wind in the Willows* is another example. 'Piper at the Gates of Dawn' (from *The Healing Game*) presents Morrison's world view in microcosm. The lyrics of the song actually quote the eponymous chapter of Grahame's book: there's wind in the willows, a piper at the gates of dawn, and everyone is listening to the silence. But one quickly spots the wider appeal of the novel to Morrison. In Grahame's parable of modern times, the quiet-living riverbank dwellers Rat and Mole see their way of life under threat from those noisy modernists, the Wild-Wooders, and the consumerist Toad. Morrison doesn't want the peace of his riverbank disturbed either. He doesn't want innovation. He wants to retain the traditional forms of existence that guarantee maintenance of the solitary quiet. His own behaviour may be as boorish as Toad's, but his philosophy and his insistently innocent message remains emphatically that of the riverbank dwellers: *No rock musicians allowed in these parts.*

The nature songs of Van Morrison seek to return not only to the past, but more especially to a point of origin, somewhere in which the kernel of a simple world can be found, and where there are sources of meaning that can uplift and explain the human condition. The lyrics are merely a vehicle with which to reach that point, and once there, they can be altered or even discarded. And in some of the most sublime moments in Morrison's art, that moment occurs when words cease to have any meaning and speaking in tongues commences. When that happens, we are well on the way to that destination of complete silence — the ultimate riposte to modernity, social etiquette and rock music.

COMPLAINTS

When Van Morrison feels put upon, which seems to be quite a lot of the time, he is not shy about telling you. As many critics, commentators, colleagues, band members, friends and fans have discovered to their cost, the singer can be an utter curmudgeon. In itself, of course, this is not so remarkable. Artists throughout history have been obsessive, private, moody as hell and occasionally very, very rude. But not many of them have sung about it.

After forty years in the music business, Morrison has a long list of people that have pissed him off, and they all feature in his songs, sometimes wearing only the thinnest of disguises. Morrison has been exploited by record company executives and managers, been lied about in the tabloid press and been the subject of more than one biographical hatchet job. With the exploitation and lies, though he doubtless takes it personally, it is really a matter of the facts of showbiz life. Record company executives and managers will rip you off if you give them the opportunity; and young, hopeful musicians are easy prey. Van learned this lesson early, but remains bitter. By much the same token, it is surely naive to expect anything from a tabloid newspaper beyond fabricated stories aimed at increasing its circulation.

The biographers, perhaps, are another matter. Here, one suspects, Morrison might share some of the culpability. Only a fan of Van Morrison's would want to write his life story in the first place, but the singer's natural suspicion makes him an unusually surly subject, and one can see how this might affect a writer's attitude.

According to Clinton Heylin, on the first page of the preface to his 2002 biography *Can You Feel the Silence?*, Morrison's lawyers were on to him within moments of his hiring a research assistant. What follows Heylin's preface is 500 pages of not quite unmitigated irritation with his subject. The author seldom misses an opportunity to make fun of Van, and while it must be admitted that the singer provides manifold opportunities for this (for example, the night he angrily stormed off stage with his guitar still plugged in, finding himself catapulted back into the spotlight), Heylin occasionally dwells on these anecdotes at the expense of Morrison's art. Indeed when it comes to discussion of the music — and there isn't so very much of that — the author is often content to quote the opinions of others.

But if it is a disappointing book, Morrison himself must share some of the responsibility. It is not so much that the singer set out to give Heylin the hardest possible time, thereby apparently fuelling the author's antagonism; after all, there is no reason why any artist should cooperate with the writing of a book he does not wish to see published. No, the fundamental reason for the singer's implication in his own literary mauling is in his musical engagement over the years with his tormentors. Morrison seems to brood on perceived injustices and then seek revenge in his songs.

The earliest example of Morrison attempting to get even in a recording studio — and to this day it remains something of a *cause célèbre* in the history of recorded sound — is the thirty-one tracks of pure rubbish he cut for Bert Berns's widow in late 1967 in order to satisfy the conditions of his contract with Bang Records. Lasting between forty-eight seconds and one minute and twenty-three seconds, these 'songs' include 'Twist and Shake', 'Shake and Roll', 'Stomp and Scream', 'Scream and Holler' and 'Jump and Thump'. Since they continue to be released and presumably sold to unsuspecting Morrison fans — on one occasion under the ironic title *Payin' Dues* — it is hard to say who in the end got more even, Morrison or Mrs Berns.

Far more typical, however, are songs such as 'The Great Deception' (from 1973's *Hard Nose the Highway*) and 'You Gotta Make it Through the World' (from *A Period of Transition*, 1977), both of which contain lyrics that offer early evidence of a trust-no-one-and-do-it-to-the-other-guy-first attitude. The subject of Morrison's ire ranges from journalists ('the myth people') and newspaper owners ('scum of the lowest degree') to other musicians ('copycats'). But broadly speaking he has three main types of complaint song: songs of defiance, songs of revenge and songs of outright whingeing.

The songs of defiance run to a basic formula: *Yes, I have been treated badly by journalists/musicians/managers/women, but I will rise above it.* In 'A Town Called Paradise', for instance, from the 1986 album *No Guru, No Method, No Teacher*, 'copycats' have 'ripped off' his words, songs and melody, but ultimately what matters is 'my relationship with you'. Then, nine years later, in *Days Like This*'s 'Raincheck', he is afflicted by less specific slings and arrows of outrageous fortune, but whatever they might be, he 'won't let the bastards grind [him] down'. In the songs of revenge, Morrison tends to deal with more specific infringements against his dignity and he comes close to naming names. For example, those 'so-called friends' mentioned in 'New Biography' (from *Back on Top*, 1999), would certainly know who they are. They are the ones who 'claim to have known [him] then' and have 'such good memories'. And then, 'on the music business scene', there are the 'vicious' and 'mean' 'big-time operators' in the song of that name on 1993's *Too Long in Exile*, two of whose names are, presumably, Berns. The songs of outright whingeing deal with how difficult it is to be a creative artist ('I'm Not Feeling it Anymore' from 1991's *Hymns to the Silence*, 'Songwriter' from *Days Like This*) and a successful public figure ('Professional Jealousy' from *Hymns*, and 'Fame' and 'Goldfish Bowl' from 2003's *What's Wrong With This Picture?*).

So what of the music that comes out of Van Morrison's hurt feelings and thirst for revenge? Perhaps the first point to make is that very few of the songs seem in any way Irish. With the exception of 'Why Must I Always Explain?', another tale of wrongdoing from the *Hymns to the Silence* double album, you will search Morrison's songs of complaint in vain for the telltale presence of uillean pipes. The sound of the pipes and the pentatonic scales that generally underpin them crop up in his songs of childhood, his love songs and his mystical songs.

Complaints

The complaining songs are about business, and business, to Van Morrison, means 'jazz, blues and funk', and most of all it means rhythm and blues. So the more bitter the song, the bluesier it tends to be.

'Underlying depression', as Morrison tells us in the song of the same name (from 1995's *Days Like This*), 'ain't nothing but the blues', and the singer's gripes, as with the blues of yore, form a starting point for musical therapy. The expression 'singing the blues' is really short for 'singing the blues *away*', and in songs, which, on the page, can seem little more than exercises in grumbling, Morrison's performances approach something akin to a vocal strut. He lifts his listeners (and himself) up, rising above his tormentors. Even when he is not employing a strict blues template (for example, on most of *Days Like This*) his voice has a blues stridency. The complaining songs are sung by Van the brawler, and he could never be mistaken for Van the mystic.

The single exception, and it is one that severely tests this rule (and the listener's patience), is 'Golden Autumn Day', the final song from *Back on Top*. The title and the tempo, the string ensemble, the gentle flick of the drums and the sweet twiddlings of Georgie Fame's Hammond organ all conspire to reassure us that we are heading once more into some 'Avalon sunset' of Van's imagining. Perhaps God will be there, too. Several of his stock catchphrases and clichés are quickly mentioned: the bells are ringing, 'the sun is shining gold', Van himself has a smile on his face and he's getting 'on with the show'. True, it turns out that this is a 'God-forsaken place', but it doesn't prevent him from soaking up another of those Indian summers and pretending he's in 'paradise', 'on a

A soul in wonder

golden autumn day'. So all is basically right in this latest garden of Eden when — would you Adam-and-Eve it? — a couple of thugs attack our man while he is parking his car.

How this happens, from a sheerly logistical point of view, is anyone's guess. Do they drag him from the vehicle as the motor is running? Do they get in the car with him? Precise use of language has never been Morrison's strong suit, so let us assume that the car parking has in fact taken place, and as he leaves the vehicle he is jumped on from behind. Van tells us that the two toughs force him to the ground and then pull a knife. But the next thing you know, our hero has 'fought [his] way up' and the two craven attackers have 'scarpered from the scene'. We can only imagine what has transpired to make the assailants give up so suddenly. (Perhaps Van growled at them.)

Meanwhile, the song itself, which is still sauntering along as though nothing untoward had occurred, dives back into a second chorus of Indian summers, paradise and golden autumn days. By the final verse, we are in Blake's 'green and pleasant' land (so it *was* Avalon after all!), but now it seems that Van has only one use for this verdant landscape. If there were any justice in the world, he harrumphs, he would be out there 'in the nearest green field' with his attackers, flogging them to within an inch of their lives. This would be a perfect 'lesson to the bleeders of the system'. The case for the restoration of public birching having been made, it is time for one more refrain about golden sunlight, as the strings gently play us out. It is hard to know what Morrison thought he was doing in this song. Perhaps it's best to regard 'Golden Autumn Day' as a minor comic masterpiece and leave it at that. Elsewhere, Van's complaining takes on a far more strident tone.

Complaints

Really, it is 'Drumshanbo Hustle' that offers the first sign of Morrison's obsessive revisiting of old grudges. Although it didn't see the light of day until the release of *The Philosopher's Stone* rarities compilation in June 1998, the song had been recorded back in 1973 around the time of *Hard Nose the Highway*, and it seems to be a direct reference to his dealings with the Bernses. They, we learn, 'were trying to muscle in' and make easy money, while 'you' (that is, Van) 'were puking up your guts' after having taken a look at 'the standard contract', which, for reasons never explained, 'you' had already signed without reading. It is hard to feel terribly sorry for the singer on this occasion, partly because he obviously should have read the contract, but mainly because he seems to have been able to turn the situation to his advantage. While Mrs Berns might have ended up with thirty-one of the worst tracks ever recorded, Morrison himself has been tapping the bitter experience for new songs ever since.

'Drumshanbo Hustle' is an up-tempo, feel-good number. Perhaps that is why it remained unreleased for a quarter of a century. Perhaps it didn't fit the bad-mood blues image that Van was cultivating in these songs.

'Big Time Operators' is far more typical of that style. Its parent album, *Too Long in Exile*, is a back-to-basics record in many ways, containing more pure r&b than any of Van's other studio releases, and even has a new version of Morrison's classic from his Them days, 'Gloria'. No wonder he got to thinking about the Bernses all over again. On 'Big Time Operators', there is the young Van in New York, where said operators are variously trying to have him 'deported', stopping him 'from getting work', blacklisting him 'all over', spreading

A soul in wonder

'malicious rumours', threatening to see him 'busted for drugs' and putting a bug in his room 'to listen in on [his] calls'. They were 'very desperate people', these big-time operators, and Morrison tells them what he thinks of them one more time, to the tune of a slow but increasingly hard-driven blues.

A decade later, on 'Goldfish Bowl', Morrison takes on a range of different pests. Ostensibly, this is a song that complains about the attention he receives because he is 'a celebrity'. And so, as in 'Songwriter', 'I'd Love to Write Another Song' (from 1989's *Avalon Sunset*) and 'Why Must I Always Explain?', the singer attempts to demystify his chosen profession. He is 'just a guy who sings songs', has neither a 'hit record' nor a 'TV show', and cannot understand why anyone should be interested in him since he has 'no reason to live in a goldfish bowl'. It is hard to escape the feeling that he protests too much about his lack of a hit record, but otherwise the thrust of his argument is plain enough: being a songwriter is like being a brain surgeon or a garbage collector; you do it to the best of your ability and that is that.

But of course that isn't that. Garbage collectors are always being complained about because they drop rubbish in the street, and brain surgeons are sued if they screw up. One is, after all, accountable for one's actions. Certainly, songwriters who do not wish to be discussed and judged should refrain from singing their songs, giving concerts and making records. What does Van Morrison want? Nodding acceptance of everything he does? No negative criticism of any sort, no analytical consideration of his work — not even too much praise? 'I'm just doing my gigs', he pleads. But if he feels like a goldfish in a bowl, perhaps he should avoid stages and spotlights.

Complaints

The crux of 'Goldfish Bowl' is its chorus. Here, for the first time in a song — and it is significant that it is one of his complaining songs — Van Morrison spells out exactly what it is he does: 'Jazz, blues and funk,' he pronounces, slowly and deliberately, as though to a small child or an idiot. 'That's *not* . . . rock . . . 'n' roll.' You sense that this is a point he has been wanting to make for quite a while, no matter that the track immediately follows an unashamedly rocking version of Lightnin' Hopkins 'Stop Drinking'. 'Folk with a beat,' Van continues, somewhat lamely, 'and a little bit of soul.' (A *little* bit of soul?)

For many reasons, this is an extremely interesting song, the centrepiece really of *What's Wrong With This Picture?*, a moderately interesting, but beautifully crafted and very well sung album. 'Goldfish Bowl' is another slow blues, a little heavier and with a distinctly hotter vocal than 'Big Time Operators', but otherwise in the same vein. Ten years on from 'Big Time Operators', however, Morrison has an extra point to prove. A matter of prestige perhaps.

What's Wrong was his first release on Blue Note, in October 2003. Although this was not the first time he'd recorded for a jazz label — in the mid 1990s *How Long Has This Been Going On* and *Tell Me Something* had both appeared on Verve — one senses from the start of the thirteen-song collection that Van is trying extra hard. Perhaps he felt he needed to live up to a label with a back catalogue including Thelonious Monk, Charlie Mingus, Jackie McLean and Gerry Mulligan (to name only some of the other Ms). Suddenly his voice seems younger and more focused than on the preceding albums, and here he is insisting that his mission in life is to sing 'jazz, blues and funk'. There is no slagging off of record company executives in 'Goldfish Bowl', possibly because Van is keen to remain on good terms with his new label, but still the 'parasites and psychic vampires' get it in the neck for 'projecting their shadow onto everyone else'. This is a flabby and unfortunate phrase, and further evidence that Morrison fails to understand that poetic imagery has to be accurate or it doesn't really mean anything. (One does not project a shadow, one *casts* it; and vampires, which, according to legend, have no shadows, can't even do that.) And more importantly, who are these 'psychic vampires'? Van seems to want to keep it vague.

This is not unusual. In fact, when one lines up all of Van Morrison's complaint songs, vagueness turns out to be a common feature. He only seems as though he is naming names. In reality, he hints, albeit rather strongly on occasion. Even mention of the Bernses is imprecise, which, given the litigious nature of that relationship, is hardly surprising. And the many references to 'copycats', 'bastards', 'hustlers', 'bleeders of the system', 'psychic vampires' and — most common of all — plain old anonymous 'they' tell us nothing at all, except that there are people out there who, Van believes, have it in for him.

Apparently, these people threaten Morrison's freedom and creativity, but more importantly in the singer's own mind they threaten his professionalism, and to a man as devoted to the Protestant work ethic as George Ivan Morrison, that is wholly unacceptable. Van is a journeyman, 'a working man in [his] prime'. He goes 'straight back to work' whether or not he is suffering from 'underlying depression' or simply 'not feeling it anymore'. He is intent on 'delivering the product on time'. Woe betide anyone who gets in his way.

The more one listens to these songs, the more it seems that Morrison is not addressing the 'bastards' and 'copycats' at all, but talking to himself. He is determined, remember, that the 'bastards' will not be allowed to 'grind [him] down'; that is the point of 'Raincheck'. Equally, in 'A Town Called Paradise', he is not overly concerned with the 'copycats', explaining that the only thing that matters is 'my relationship with you'. Could this 'you' be us, his audience? And is he using his irritation with the 'copycats', 'bastards', 'hustlers' and 'psychic vampires', harnessing it, like energy, in order to 'write [*us*] another song'?

Yet it is just when Morrison proclaims his professional credentials most stridently that we find him on shaky ground. Take 'Songwriter', from *Days Like This*. Here he tells us again and again that songwriting is his job. He does it 'for a living', he writes 'about men and women'; he can 'do it for certain' and even when he's 'hurtin''. Maybe. But 'Songwriter' is a terrible song. In fact, if this song were a typical example of his work, he would have starved to death. It has a dreary tune and the words seem to be almost deliberately bad. One pauses, momentarily, to wonder if Morrison is being ironic — but it doesn't seem likely.

What this piece offers, paradoxically, is stark evidence that Morrison is not a 'songwriter' at all, not in the sense that, say, Bob Dylan, Randy Newman and Burt Bacharach are. His songs are not routinely sung by others, and that is because as words and music on the page the vast majority of them are surprisingly ordinary. For every 'Moondance', there are dozens more compositions that no one but Van would want to sing.

A soul in wonder

The songs often fail on the page, because so few of them have anything approaching a literary structure. Dylan writes narrative songs that tell stories ('Desolation Row', 'Tangled Up in Blue', 'Isis' and a hundred others) or dissect a relationship in detail ('Like a Rolling Stone', 'If You See Her Say Hello'), things that Morrison's can't do because the majority of them lack the linearity required to make such an exposition or present an argument. From the point of view of the lyrics, Morrison's songs tend to be a rough assemblage of images and references — fascinating, to be sure, but not, on their own, especially cogent. What holds them together and what gives them meaning and sometimes greatness is the way Morrison sings them.

That voice is the heart of the matter. Time and again, Morrison's songs, whichever of the above categories they seem to fit, resist our attempts to fathom their precise literary allusions and philosophical preoccupations simply because they exist in the world of sound. You understand a Van Morrison song not when you read it, but when you hear him sing it. So let's go back to the beginning and listen.

PART TWO

A working man in his prime

NOTHING BUT A STRANGER IN THIS WORLD (1968–1974)

■ *Astral Weeks* ■ *Moondance* ■ *His Band and the Street Choir* ■ *Tupelo Honey* ■ *Saint Dominic's Preview* ■ *Hard Nose the Highway* ■ *Veedon Fleece*

The history of artistic achievement is littered with examples of expatriation leading to the creation of identifiably local artefacts, with the homeland often being seen more clearly from a foreign perspective. James Joyce's Dublin epic *Ulysses* was written in Zurich, Trieste and Paris, while Frederick Delius's pastoral English tone-poems were coloured by the composer's experiences in a Florida orange orchard and later in France. In Australia, orchestral composers only began to write in distinctive nationalist idioms after encountering Indonesian and Japanese music. Through working in foreign environments, these artists gained new insight into the nature and character of their own culture and national identity.

A working man in his prime

In the case of the Ulsterman Van Morrison, the overwhelming influence has always been American music. But while that quiet obsession with the music of his youth remains unchanged over a four-decade career, Morrison's encounters with American culture have been simultaneously profound and difficult. Like generations of Irishmen before him, Morrison — especially during the early part of his career — had to come to terms with the power of an American culture that could have swallowed him up as an original artist. The story of how it didn't, but rather of how it nourished him and made him into the unique and instantly recognisable 'voice' he is today, reveals a heroic side to an artist more often associated with intuitive and naive inspiration than the struggle for identity.

Although Van didn't end up emigrating to America as planned when his father looked to make a new life there for the family in the 1950s, his life at home in Belfast was imbued with its culture. Morrison's first trip to the United States, then, was in the heyday of his band Them. And after the group's break-up he would work there again with the creator of 'Here Comes the Night', Bert Berns, on some potential singles (including 'T.B. Sheets', 'Brown Eyed Girl' and other works subsequently collected under the title *Blowin' Your Mind*). But these were fleeting visits, and despite comparative success in the American Top 40 with some of these early pieces, nothing could have prepared Morrison fully for his eventual long-term move to the United States in 1968.

From that time until late 1973, Morrison would not return at all to the land of his birth. Instead, he set up home in Woodstock, New York, and then moved on to Fairfax,

Nothing but a stranger in this world (1968–1974)

California, before a brief holiday in Ireland resulted in a profound artistic reorientation that, in hindsight, seems had been brewing all along. The period from 1968 to 1974 would represent the most concentrated phase of Morrison's career, during which he would release his first seven solo albums and pursue his career essentially as an 'American artist'. And as the following analysis of those extraordinary first solo albums demonstrates, that musical and personal journey within America, book-ended by the albums *Astral Weeks* on one side and *Veedon Fleece* on the other, resulted not so much in the 'Americanisation' of Van Morrison as in his rediscovery of his 'Irishness'. These early solo records redefined him — not so much as a musician but as an individual — and set up the themes that would sustain virtually the entirety of his subsequent oeuvre.

The journey traced during this first phase of Morrison's solo career has a distinctly geographical character in its themes and imaginative orientation, not to mention in Morrison's own place of residence. With each new album release, figuratively he moved further west through America, assimilating wherever possible to his new culture until, in California in the early 1970s, he could go no further, reaching a cultural impasse and an artistic crisis.

But for great artists, crises of identity are the challenges that are overcome during the achievement of creative triumph. Responding to an America that was more about great deceptions and big-time operators rather than the Wild West heroes and good-versus-bad moral battles of his boyhood imagining, Morrison in his twenties turned out seven albums that even today, despite their momentary lapses in standards,

A working man in his prime

remain at the pinnacle of popular music achievement. Inadvertently they narrate a personal struggle and an adventure into the American frontier as compelling as anything in a Zane Grey novel.

ASTRAL WEEKS
(November 1968)

- *Astral Weeks* ▪ *Beside You* ▪ *Sweet Thing* ▪ *Cyprus Avenue* ▪ *The Way Young Lovers Do* ▪ *Madame George* ▪ *Ballerina* ▪ *Slim Slow Slider*

Recorded at New York's Century Sound studios with both white American and African–American musicians, and with its lyrics infused with not-so-distant memories of a Belfast childhood, *Astral Weeks* encapsulates virtually all the major preoccupations and themes that would sustain Van Morrison's subsequent career. It is an album about innocence and experience where, in the contradictory voice of the ancient Mississippi bluesman, the young singer depicts himself caught amid the world of childlike wonder. The prison and the chain-gang and the boozy, sultry nights in bars that are the stuff of the original musical inspiration are here replaced by the purity of childlike visions and the wonder of a prelapsarian world. Whether intentionally or not, it's Blakean, the nursery-school lyrics containing the growls and grumbles of a diabolical sensibility.

But most of all, *Astral Weeks* is an album that dreams of the rivers and the railways of Ulster, the viaducts and the avenues, all of them geographic pathways out of town and all of them

Nothing but a stranger in this world (1968–1974)

equally the means through which the imagination can be freed. In his later work, Morrison would reminisce and want to be taken back to those childhood days, but in this, his first foray into the depths of his Irish aesthetic, *Astral Weeks* is looking for a way out. Far from the nostalgic album that Morrison would later make a speciality — and in spite of its constant references to those heady days of spiritual intoxication in 1950s Belfast — *Astral Weeks* is all about journeying far from home. It's about going out into the world, discovering new things, and finding a land of wonder.

Morrison uses Belfast as his point of reference for a far-from-home reflection on the modern European diaspora. More than anything else, *Astral Weeks* is an album fixated on alienation and expatriation. Quite fittingly then, the session musicians assembled by Morrison and producer Lewis Merenstein — drummer Connie Kay from the Modern Jazz Quartet, percussionist Warren Smith Jr, session guitarist Jay Berliner, ex–Miles Davis bassist Richard Davis, and flautist/saxophonist John Payne — were personal and musical strangers.

Given that music can never be explicitly programmatic, the opening, title track of *Astral Weeks* nevertheless begins with an all-pervading sense of momentum that can only be suggestive of some distant journey into unknown territory. Where are we going? There is an urgency in those opening bars prefacing the singer's entry, as if the players are simply hanging on for the thrilling ride. And hang on they must.

There is enough historical information concerning the two-and-a-bit *Astral Weeks* sessions of September and October 1968 to suggest a more literal interpretation of musicians hanging on in unchartered territory. But this reality only contributes to the

A working man in his prime

musical outcome — for us as listeners, and them as players fumbling through half-written, barely understood charts — of going somewhere unknown.

The lyrics are largely unintelligible; we are venturing 'in the slipstream, between the viaducts of your dream', but wherever we're headed, it seems that only the singer can be the guide. Over the course of the track, one practically hears bass player Richard Davis catching on and working out where he is, throwing in experimental blues notes to ground it, with the other instruments then progressively falling into line. But really, from the entry of the vocal, the song 'Astral Weeks' actually becomes an extended *rallentando*, winding its way down to 'another time . . . another place', the violins shimmering like an aeroplane engine cutting back as landing approaches. And at last the slowing becomes exaggerated. We are at our destination.

Despite the elegant intro to 'Beside You', Jay Berliner exchanging the previous track's folk-rock lead for a more fluent, hybrid of Spanish guitar and blues, the instruments in Morrison's session band wander around with a hint of style but a little desperation too in the album's second track. And like Dylan with his baffled country musicians on that notorious, caffeine-fuelled, semi-improvised take on 'Sad-Eyed Lady of the Lowlands' (*Blonde on Blonde*), Morrison's penetrating, clarion call of a voice provides the only stable centre in this new world.

The search for meaning has begun, and in hesitant rhythm, the emigrants fan out across the plains. In this, the second version of the song (like 'Madame George', it was one of the tracks recorded for Bang Records the previous year),

Nothing but a stranger in this world (1968–1974)

'Beside You' holds together magnificently, but on a purely technical level, the ensemble work on this and other tracks from *Astral Weeks* must qualify as some of the loosest playing ever recorded on disc.

The tempo picks up again for 'Sweet Thing', the yearning strings of 'Astral Weeks' returning and Connie Kay's drum kit making its first appearance (albeit, only the hi-hats). The sense of rebirth is palpable, from the opening where the protagonist drinks — for the first but by no means the last time in Morrison's oeuvre — from the clear water, on to the gardens 'wet with rain'. In this New World, which two songs back seemed so strange, and one song ago could barely accommodate life, the source of hope and sustenance emerges. Here is a young man, having pulled himself together, now let off the leash and running for his creative life. And in an echo — whether conscious or unconscious — of Dylan's 'My Back Pages', the young man protests that he 'will never grow so old again'. In fact he will. The May Day images and ideas about rebirth and rejuvenation underlying 'Sweet Thing' will recur frequently throughout the next three decades of Morrison's career.

We are hearing an 'Irish' album of course, but in the middle of it, as the New World is surveyed, the aesthetic is perhaps more akin to Walt Whitman. In 'Cyprus Avenue', the tempo slows again as we ponder random impressions drawn from ordinary life. In a precursor to the work of Bruce Springsteen (and one of the initial indications to justify Van's complaint that Springsteen 'ripped me off'), we are in a world where from our car seat we ponder 'the mansion on the hill'. But Van's roving eye soon settles on what will also become a familiar topic in his subsequent career: appreciation of little girls on their way back home from school.

As he will continue to do right through until the blistering live version of 'Good Morning Little Schoolgirl' from 1994's *A Night in San Francisco*, the mere thought of jailbait turns this spiritual seeker into a stuttering, tongue-tied mess. Best to try to forget about forbidden fruit and instead go wandering down by the railway tracks, where the spirit of the Beat poets accompany the searcher on one side, and the folk traditions in which girls have rainbow ribbons in their hair stroll by on the other. Again it's like Whitman's vision of the fledgling America, filled with catalogues of observances, common sights and objects invested with a new, foreign character through the alienation of a European eye (and an Irish memory) within an American landscape.

It's a disjointed, impressionistic vision, and the sound-world of 'Cyprus Avenue', in which harpsichord and violin are prominent, makes the sense of estrangement all the more disconcerting and wonderful. It becomes an avenue of dreams, and just as in the opening title track, when it all begins to get out of hand — with Davis's bass still not seeming to know what to play — it 'lands' again, slowing down into the fade-out. We're now at the halfway mark of what Van originally conceived as an 'opera', and side one, the quasi-biblical 'In the beginning' section, has just ended. The Old Testament tales of creation and exodus are completed; the world of Babylon and hedonism are just a flipside away.

When we begin 'Afterwards', there's a swinging party going on. Horn- and vibraphone-heavy, the big-band feel of 'The Way Young Lovers Do' takes the form of a combined

Nothing but a stranger in this world (1968–1974)

sacred and profane dance. This is Aubrey Beardsley territory, with whirling dervishes and strangled, mangled horn squawks. Never a great mover himself, this song inaugurates Morrison's career-long fascination with the dance, but more importantly, it sets up a frantic sound-world from which the album's truly immortal track, 'Madame George', can emerge.

Throughout this extraordinary album, Morrison's voice is always the prophetic guiding light, and never more so than on this three-chord wonder of a song, with its guided tour of idyllic East Belfast childhood haunts. There is an ominous military bearing to the accompaniment, with the mechanical guitar-strumming and Kay's side-drum rat-a-tat suddenly introducing structure and order to replace the free-form improvisations that have melted the bar-lines of tracks on the previous side of the album.

The languid accompaniment to 'Madame George' is acoustic but that searing voice is electric, clashing and impassioned as it nevertheless sinks into a trance. We're on the train again, and only Van knows where it's going — quite literally, seeing as no one else playing on the album would ever have heard of Sandy Row. Stream-of-consciousness memories recall 'the rain, hail, sleet and snow', while kid stuff drifts over Morrison's mental horizon — throwing pennies from the bridges. (A similar litany of childhood recollections surfaces in Tom Waits's glorious 'Kentucky Avenue'.)

And eventually, as the transcendent moment arrives, for the first time in his career, Van begins to speak in tongues as the hypnotic, meaningless mantra 'To love to loves to love to loves' transports the entire argument into the non-verbal realm. Not long after this album's release, George Harrison would begin chanting 'Hare Krishna, hare rama' in hit songs and Jim Morrison was extemporising doggerel for fifteen minutes at a time, but no other pop musician so convincingly entered into an altered spiritual state as Van does on this improvised journey into someplace else.

And for the next thirty-five years, sometimes when Morrison was in inspired mood — in 'Listen to the Lion' (from *Saint Dominic's Preview*), for instance, or 'In the Garden' (*No Guru, No Method, No Teacher*), and even at moments during *A Night in San Francisco* — he would approach this hypnotic space of 'Madame George' again. The rest of the time he was either trying desperately and unsuccessfully to find it, or pretending that he didn't care anymore. He cared. He still cares. And why wouldn't he? The song remains as close to perfection as he or virtually anyone else in pop has ever come. Not a bad effort considering he never really knew if he was singing about Joy or George.

The fade-out to 'Madame George', where the tempo picks up with momentary urgency as the vocal line of 'Say goodbye, goodbye' wails over the top, would re-emerge later in the work of Bruce Springsteen. Each time in altered but recognisable form, Springsteen used it to shape the similarly triumphant conclusions to 'Thunder Road', 'Jungleland' and, most of all, the title track on *Born to Run*. With his acute musical ear, the Boss learned from Van Morrison and 'Madame George' just how convincing it can be when the coda, in rapture, waves an awestruck goodbye to the mystical, self-sufficient world of a great song.

The transition to 'Ballerina' (which some critics find unconvincing) represents the first non-change of tempo

Nothing but a stranger in this world (1968–1974)

between tracks on the album. It's another slow guitar-strum with loose, even sloppy accompaniment. Of course, after the miracle of 'Madame George', anything is going to sound like a disappointment. For all its suffering in comparison, 'Ballerina' features an astonishing vocal from Morrison, practically screaming some of the time, and even the violin fills out the texture and flicks the momentum switch effectively on the line 'Well, I may be wrong'. In a reversal of the trend from the earlier part of the album, 'Ballerina' speeds up towards the end and there's a sense of taking off. But we're only going as far as Ladbroke Grove — in Belfast, not London — for the next song.

'Slim Slow Slider' enters in cruisy mode and with a sense of resolution. The alien has adapted to his new landscape and Van even has the temerity to laugh during his vocalising! Payne's squealing soprano sax is prominent (a foreshadowing of the oboe lines on *No Guru, No Method, No Teacher*) and genuinely echoes and embellishes the singing, unlike much of his flute playing on the album. But no sooner has the song established itself than producer Lewis Merenstein pulls a masterstroke, making a massive cut in the recorded take as suddenly the tempo picks up like a piece of paper caught in a whirlwind. Within seconds, this entire, elaborately created new world of wonder is simply swept into the ether. The stranger in a strange land has quit while he's ahead, and the technique of all good tragedies of alienation, expatriation, innocence and experience is employed, as the rest is left to silence.

Although it was surely never intended, *Astral Weeks* now seems like a manifesto, a statement of intent: *This is the kind*

A working man in his prime

of artist I am, and this is what I will remain. In 1968, when Morrison's peers were either donning denim suits and inventing the blues-based 'rock' idiom, or adding pedal-steel guitars and 'going country', this was pop music born again.

MOONDANCE
(February 1970)

▪ *And It Stoned Me* ▪ *Moondance* ▪ *Crazy Love* ▪ *Caravan* ▪ *Into the Mystic* ▪ *Come Running* ▪ *These Dreams of You* ▪ *Brand New Day* ▪ *Everyone* ▪ *Glad Tidings*

Only fourteen months elapsed between the release of *Astral Weeks* and the arrival of *Moondance* but they seem worlds apart and from different eras. In a very real sense they were, for that short intervening period was a tumultuous time in history. The impact of the student demonstrations of 1968 was felt around the world, as was the democratic uprising in Prague and its subsequent violent Communist suppression. The Vietnam War raged and Neil Armstrong landed on the moon.

In Morrison's native Belfast, the Troubles had begun, with the city that the singer had just depicted as the location of an idyllic youth now more segregated and murderous than ever. In popular culture, the epoch-making festivals at Woodstock, Isle of Wight and (less so) Altamont heralded possibilities for a new age of Aquarius, but by late 1970, those decade-defining Liverpudlians the Beatles had split and three figureheads of the youth movement — Brian Jones, Jimi Hendrix and Janis Joplin — would all be dead. The transition

Nothing but a stranger in this world (1968–1974)

from the 1960s to the '70s was therefore much more momentous than the simple passing of one year into another. It marked the end of one era — and one state of mind — and the beginning of another.

Musically, Morrison had entered into the world of his Woodstock near-neighbours, the Band, with their tight ensemble and stylistic melange of country-rock and r&b. The meditative, hypnotic mood of *Astral Weeks* disappeared almost as quickly as it had emerged. No more of the unique, consistent sound-world and prevailing mystical rapture that permeates *Astral Weeks*, instead Morrison turned out an album that today probably remains the most diverse stylistically of his entire career. True, there are still plenty of 'mood pieces' on *Moondance*, but those moods swing rapidly from track to track and the album is sustained not by an overriding aesthetic so much as by a string of great three- and four-minute pop songs.

It might have been recorded in New York like its predecessor, but in terms of its creative content and imaginative landscape, *Moondance* actually depicts Morrison setting sail from his native Belfast, bound for America. At the beginning of the album, he's still the Belfast child of *Astral Weeks*, recalling a fishing expedition near the county fair. By the middle, however, he's embarked on a series of journeys, on foot, on a boat, in a gypsy caravan, heading spiritually into the mystic and imaginatively into a brand new day. By album's end, he has arrived, sending greetings back home from his new base in New York. In short, where *Astral Weeks* captures the mystical moment of transcendence, *Moondance* traces the geographical journey that gives rise to it.

A working man in his prime

Still, those distinctive 'moments in time' remain, right from the opening track 'And It Stoned Me'. It sounds like a song the Band might have recorded on their groundbreaking album *Music From Big Pink*, and certainly Morrison's new ensemble (assembled especially for these sessions in late 1969) has a definite sense of slick professionalism about it. Throughout the album, the players are tight and focused, guitarist John Platania, keyboard player Jeff Labes and saxophonist Jack Schroer regularly taking solos, assembling the first component parts of what would eventually become one of Morrison's best bands, the Caledonia Soul Orchestra. Other contributors to *Moondance*, both of whom would also become regular sidemen during this period, included the rhythm section of Gary Malabar (on drums and vibraphone) and John Klingberg (bass).

'And It Stoned Me' is a typical Morrison nature-worship song, beginning with the rain pouring down in the first line and leading up to the moment where — as in the previous album's 'Sweet Thing' — the singer stoops down to collect the water from the mountain stream. The direct experience of the environment creates a natural high, which Morrison equates to the sexual act, referring to it for the first time as 'jellyroll' (a stock blues euphemism with a variety of sexual connotations). There's a curious quality to Morrison's voice on this track. He's in fine form but the recorded sound has a flangey quality to it, as if he were singing the vocals through a megaphone, or the voice was coming out stridently from some distant past. And that's one of the features of the *Moondance* album generally: the voice sounds different on virtually every track.

Nothing but a stranger in this world (1968–1974)

The title track, which comes next, remains an exceptional moment in Morrison's career. While it is, without doubt, his best-known song, its poppy lounge-jazz feel is atypical of his songwriting. Of course Morrison has always flirted with jazz, and indeed has made explicitly 'jazz' albums (including 1995's *How Long Has This Been Going On*), but few would claim that he has any natural affinity with the style. It is difficult to name even one other song from his forty-year career that manages to capture the jazz-pop feel remotely as well as 'Moondance'.

Just where the appeal of this widely covered hit resides is also difficult to describe. The prevailing image of dancing in the moonlight is romantic and sensual enough, but it's hardly strikingly original. The instrumental playing is adequate, even if Colin Tilton's shrill flute obbligato risks drowning out the vocal. But the track works, quite simply, because it swings. There is a natural flow to the repeated two-chord pattern, and the partial walking-bass and syncopations only serve to highlight the song's easy groove. And then of course there is the voice, at its most penetrating and pure, resolving towards the end into the gargle of an outboard-motor effect.

Like much jazz, 'Moondance' feels like a lifestyle as well as a tune. It's one of those tracks that simply leaps out at you and is almost impossible not to like. After the comparative obscurity and navel-gazing of much of the *Astral Weeks* set, the 24-year-old Van Morrison had created a hit for the ages.

Next up, 'Crazy Love' is perhaps not so impressive a song, but its vocal quality is equally remarkable, featuring a bizarre, strangely appealing use of Morrison's head voice. Normally, Van's vocals are among the most distinctive in the pop genre, and this would be probably the only song in which his voice — on being heard 'cold' — could prove unrecognisable. It's Morrison in weasel/choirboy mode, falsetto and insipid in a song in which the real sense of soul comes not from the frontman but from the back-up singers (which include Cissy Houston). The call-and-response routine between them is the first hint of true gospel in Morrison's work, and an early indication of the artist adapting to his new American environment.

Jeff Labes then plays two emphatic piano trills leading to a perfunctory chord, after which the keyboard descends into the unmistakeable groove of 'Caravan', one of the truly great Van Morrison songs. The sense of journey is all-pervasive. Here, Morrison indulges what would prove to be an enduring obsession with gypsies, while, right from the start of the brilliant live version (subsequently released on *It's Too Late To Stop Now*), employing a typically opaque use of language in the form of repeated 'mama mama, look at Emma Rose' stutters and the pivotal calls of 'La la la-la, la-la la'.

As the radio blares out from the distance and the campfire roars, 'Caravan' becomes a catalogue of Morrison's early themes — the outdoor life, a never-ending journey, folk culture bringing a sense of community, and the restorative power of a simple rural existence. In keeping with this, the steady chord progression provides plenty of opportunity for improvisation and solos, which Morrison and his various bands have always grasped in live performances of the song. (An excellent version is also captured on *The Last Waltz*, Martin Scorsese's documentary of the Band's farewell concert in November 1976.)

Nothing but a stranger in this world (1968–1974)

The journey metaphor continues on the next track, but now with an ecstatic-sounding Van 'borne before the wind' out on the ocean. 'Into the Mystic' is another Morrison classic, both musically strong and incorporating key elements of the artist's style and themes. Aside from these attributes, the use of the song's final line — 'It's too late to stop now' — as the title of his first live album would ensure a greater status for 'Into the Mystic' than mere album track. (Ten years later, the tune would also serve as a walk-on theme for his second live set, *Live at the Grand Opera House, Belfast*.)

Whereas 'Caravan' draws its literary meaning from nineteenth-century English pastoral literature (such as Matthew Arnold's 'The Scholar Gipsy' and George Borrow's book *Lavengro*), 'Into the Mystic' taps into an even richer tradition, where the sea journey is symbolic of a spiritual quest. Originally, Morrison intended it to be a journey into the 'misty' ocean, but eventually opted for the more literary, more resonant choice of diction. The gypsy is still with him in 'Into the Mystic' — in the form of the lover's soul that he intends to 'rock' — but this time the wandering gypsies actually have three points of destination. One, of course, is sexual conquest (the rocking is not just of the boat!), and the consequent transformation 'into the mystic' has a decidedly carnal element: sexual nirvana awaits if the lover comes with him. But, more spiritually, the wind as the force of nature is blowing Van out into the wide blue yonder, where the mystic can 'float' magnificently within the transcendental space so familiar from *Astral Weeks*. And thirdly, there is the homecoming sense of the mystical. But interestingly, while the 'foghorn' referred to in the song's bridge sections could at a literal level merely announce

A working man in his prime

the return of the sea-gypsy to his home port (identified by literal-minded critics as Belfast), in terms of the whole lyric, 'home' is actually the mystical state rather than any specific geographic location. When Van Morrison comes home, he does so to a world of spiritual calm — what he would subsequently describe on 1980's *Common One* album as a 'haunt of ancient peace'. Belfast, blowing itself up in civil war in 1970, is no longer his true home. It would be another four years before Morrison, on *Veedon Fleece*, would actually associate his home in the spiritual dimension with any kind of national Irish identity. On the contrary, at this stage of his career, the sailor protagonist of 'Into the Mystic' is heading towards a home that is beyond the reach of maps, beyond the horizon, and if ever a landmass does loom into view, it's more likely going to be America than his country of origin.

In successive tracks, we've had the gypsy caravan, then the 'bonnie' boat, and now in 'Come Running' we're down at the railway line, such a common setting for American blues and r&b songs. 'By the side of the tracks where the train goes by', to be precise, the sound of a conga drum adding to the idea of carriages rattling over the rails. And of course, there's wind and rain, which will force the object of devotion to 'come running' to Van, who in turn promises satisfaction 'in the morning sun'. A bright, simple shuffle, 'Come Running' places the album firmly back on (albeit wet) land — and more particularly within the world of American pop. Logically then, this was the song chosen as a radio-friendly first single off *Moondance*.

On the original, vinyl format of the album, 'Come Running' was located at the beginning of side two, and the

Nothing but a stranger in this world (1968–1974)

orientation is now American through and through. Indeed if 'executive producer' Lewis Merenstein (Morrison having taken production credit this time around) had had the opportunity to name the two sides as he did on *Astral Weeks*, he might have done worse than 'Flight from Ireland' and 'Arrival in America'. It's now a critical commonplace that the second half of *Moondance* is weaker than the first — not surprising given the consistent, arguably never-to-be-bettered strength of the album's first side — but it's more a question of an aesthetic shift than a weakening of inspiration. With his band humming along behind him like a well-tuned internal combustion engine, on side two Van has set out for the bright lights of America and is revelling in a paradise of musical styles and genres now freely at his disposal.

And once he's there, his thoughts turn to moving on still further, to Canada, the very first reference in 'These Dreams of You'. Considering the singer is being knocked around by the lover in the song, physically and emotionally, it's a surprisingly light-hearted and jaunty little number. In a far cry from his later songs of betrayal and complaint, Van even seems to regard the person smacking him in the chops as 'an angel sent down from above'. Evidently everything in America had a rosy glow for him back then, and within that context his name-checking of musical heroes (following on from Leadbelly on *Astral Weeks*) continues with soon-to-become perennial favourite Ray Charles, who, we're told, was criticised but still 'got up to do his best'. Just as the entire *Astral Weeks* album was about expatriation and alienation, tracks like 'These Dreams of You' show the immigrant singer beginning to adapt to his surroundings, trying to become more American than the Americans.

A working man in his prime

This New World theme continues in 'Brand New Day', a track that features the return of the gospel chorus. Surely one of the most underrated songs in the entire Morrison oeuvre, 'Brand New Day' takes as its theme the nineteenth-century, Whitmanesque notion of 'the American Adam', where the alienated individual who's been lost — 'used, confused and so abused' — celebrates the new day, the New World, the infinite range of possibilities now at his disposal. There can be few more optimistic or unselfconsciously uplifting songs in all Morrison's music.

Apparently inspired by having heard a song by the Band on a Boston radio station (either Dylan's 'I Shall Be Released' or, an original, the Robbie Robertson–penned 'The Weight') 'Brand New Day' is almost a paean of thanks as the rain, which has poured down from track one of the album, is blown away and the sun begins to shine. There's freedom, brightness and light once more, and the railroad track where he'd been 'shoved out' is a thing of the past. With the singer's eyes hooked on 'that beautiful morning sun', 'Brand New Day' contributes a crucial dimension to an album that not only reconciles the singer to his adopted land, but does so with an unforced ecstasy that he would never exceed during the next thirty-five years of his career.

Of course, happiness is not always a good thing for a naturally surly Celtic artist and the equally celebratory 'Everyone', which follows, sounds just a touch too cheesy thanks to Jeff Labes's bustling clavinet and the chirrupy, tuneless flute. It's like something that might be sung at a revivalist meeting when 'Kumbaya' just doesn't quite swing enough. Nevertheless, for all its moments of embarrassment,

Nothing but a stranger in this world (1968–1974)

'Everyone' locks itself into what was fast becoming Morrison's grand tradition of songs beginning down on the avenue and then progressing to a spot by a stream where the singer is able to dream — happily, given the ham-fisted rhyme scheme. Still, Van does seem more convincing as a loner than as a singalong leader, a fact borne out by much of the content of his next release, *His Band and the Street Choir*.

The boppy mood continues into the concluding 'Glad Tidings', a song seemingly inspired by a letter to the New York–based Morrison from a friend offering 'greetings from London'. The recipient of Morrison's own 'glad tidings from New York' is, like the singer himself in the middle of the *Moondance* album, in transit, but by the end of this truly joyful (and in the context of later albums, most uncharacteristic) song, it's clear that the writer is utterly comfortable at last in his new surroundings. The morning mood of 'Brand New Day' has prevailed. Now, as he lies down 'low and easy' in the American evening, perhaps in preparation for another 'moondance', there is a peace and contentment in the singer's world — and a sense of happiness in his immediate location that he would try to recreate many times in the future.

Beginning in the wet, rainy countryside of Northern Ireland with a fishing rod in his hand and tackle on his back, and ending up in a decidedly urban New York evening surrounded by businessmen, *Moondance* traces a massive geographic and emotional journey that is like an ecstatic homecoming. But as time and many more albums would prove, Morrison's restless spirit kept travelling, and New York would prove to be only a momentary resting place on a long journey.

A working man in his prime

HIS BAND AND THE STREET CHOIR
(November 1970)

▪ *Domino* ▪ *Crazy Face* ▪ *Give Me a Kiss* ▪ *I've Been Working* ▪ *Call Me Up in Dreamland* ▪ *I'll Be Your Lover Too* ▪ *Blue Money* ▪ *Virgo Clowns* ▪ *Gypsy Queen* ▪ *Sweet Jannie* ▪ *If I Ever Needed Someone* ▪ *Street Choir*

The musicians who worked on *His Band and the Street Choir* attest to the endless road trips between upstate Woodstock and A&R Recording in New York City during the sessions for this, Van Morrison's third solo album. The well-worn path would see the return of Platania, Schroer and Klingberg from the previous album — on lead guitar, horns and bass respectively — while among the new recruits was drummer Dahaud Shaar (aka David Shaw), who, to his considerable mystification, would find himself credited on the sleeve as 'assistant producer'. But while the highways of upstate New York got the band into the groove musically, the star of the show was beginning to turn his attention to the West.

California had often been a place where significant events occurred in Morrison's life. Four years earlier, for instance, Them had imploded forever while on tour in the western state. Around the same time, he met Janet Planet there. During the sessions for this album, Morrison's successful gigs at the legendary Fillmore in San Francisco created considerable interest in his music. Van was suddenly big in California, then, and not long after the clumsily titled *His Band and the Street Choir* was released, he would move there to live.

Nothing but a stranger in this world (1968–1974)

Most of all, in terms of the influence on his songwriting, the constant road trips through New York and the cross-country flights to Californian gigs meant that the post-*Moondance* Morrison was becoming an acclimatised American. The tales of expatriation and alienation that had given *Astral Weeks* and *Moondance* their substance had now been replaced by an entirely different point of view. No longer a place to go to, America was where he was, and there are few Morrison albums that maintain an American focus as clearly and consistently as this strange, often infuriating compilation of three-minute wonders from the latter part of 1970.

It's a grand tour of American popular styles built around standard twelve-bar blues ('Give Me a Kiss', 'Blue Money', 'Sweet Jannie') and extraordinarily convincing impersonations of Wilson Pickett ('Domino', 'I've Been Working'), all of it resolving into the gospel-tinged final numbers, 'If I Ever Needed Someone' and 'Street Choir'. Bob Dylan and the Band might have cast their long shadows over Morrison's earlier albums, but on this work, which was originally inspired by acappella singing on American street corners, the influence is almost all black. Horn-heavy throughout and, like *Moondance*, with a stronger first side, it has a feeling of spontaneity — too much so at times, especially when Morrison takes to the saxophone in arguably the worst playing of that instrument in his entire career.

The only 'Irish' reference on the album is an incidental one, 'Derry down green' being the 'color' (US spelling, naturally) of his dream in 'I'll Be Your Lover Too'. Instead we find the first truly ubiquitous signs of an emerging wordless Van in the spirit of 'Be bop a lula', *His Band and the Street*

Choir being notable for its nonsense lyrics and opaque repetitions of soul phrases. The abundance of 'uh-huh's, 'all right's, 'do-wop's, 'woman's, 'baby's and 'do-do-you-do's in the printed lyrics makes for painful reading.

The words, when they do emerge, are appropriately banal and clichéd, with some of the worst rhymes he would ever write in his career. Not that Morrison totally abandons his usual preoccupations in the interests of a lowest-common-denominator, radio-format LP. Instead, he employs his favoured themes as ingredients within the formula, and effectively so. Right from the outset, the Morrison motifs are there: the desire to hear rhythm-and-blues music on the radio (repeat, 'on the radio, on the radio') in 'Domino'; the lovers walking hand-in-hand down the lane as the rain threatens in 'Give Me a Kiss'; the blue-collar r&b statement of the Protestant work ethic that is 'I've Been Working', with sex the reward at the end of a long hard day; the reprisal of *Moondance*'s public-transport fixation on 'Call Me Up in Dreamland' ('from the airport to the plane' and then 'away to the railroad trains'); the gypsy of 'Gypsy Queen'; the schoolgirl reference in 'Sweet Jannie', and the singer's desire to have her come walking 'in the clear moonlight'.

This time though, rather than being the subject of the songs themselves, these characteristic Morrison motifs are incidental, part of the very fabric of the hits designed to be consumed by the masses, independent of any effort to create the mystical, hypnotic trance in which they first emerged. Where *Astral Weeks* sought to beguile with its tales of a Belfast childhood, now just two years later, *His Band and the Street Choir* whoops and hollers its way through a string of

Nothing but a stranger in this world (1968–1974)

radio-friendly lollipops. This not to say that it's a bad album as such (although Morrison himself admitted to being disappointed with it), but clearly it was put out to serve a purpose for a man who was beginning to headline at the Fillmore. Where much of the sessions that became *Blowin' Your Mind*, his previous trivial effort, had been half-hearted in their intentions, commercially cynical even, this was a genuine attempt to make engaging, workable music for the masses.

All of which is to say that in this album, the newly settled Van, with loving support and inspiration from his American wife and American-born infant daughter, Shana, attempted to put together a disc full of commercial hits that his new compatriots would buy by the truckload. And he nearly succeeded in his ambition. 'Domino', the first single, hit number 9, 'Blue Money' cracked the Top 30, and 'Call Me Up in Dreamland' also made the charts.

The album's opener, 'Domino' is a curious track in which the singer protests that he wants to hear rhythm and blues yet what he actually delivers is straight soul — horns and all — over John Platania's infectious, syncopated guitar lick. Like something out of Alan Parker's film *The Commitments*, the song finds Morrison delving into his kit-bag of soul lingo, with enough 'Lord have mercy's, 'dig it's, 'all right's and (unanswered) 'say it again's to fill an entire black American album. Its hit qualities, however, are unquestionable.

In the ballad 'Crazy Face', he's into the *John Wesley Harding* territory of American mythology (the one moment, perhaps, where Dylan and the Band make their influence felt, if only in the lyrics). Van's combination of toastmaster speech and rock screaming fails to distract from what is presumably a saxophone solo, although its strangled reed effects sound nothing like that instrument. It's a gunslinger's song, and with the reference to Jesse James it becomes apparent that, as a one-time Irish youth wearing his cowboy outfit, this was the disoriented identity-crisis lyric that Van Morrison was always destined to write. (And it wouldn't be the last of such Irish–American cowboy lyrics either, with 'Linden Arden Stole the Highlights' and 'Who Was That Masked Man?' appearing on 1974's *Veedon Fleece*.)

Next up is 'Give Me a Kiss', where Morrison's wordlessness now extends to 'do-doot n' do-dit, do-dit, do-dit's and 'do-wop's. This track could have come from any American bar-band of the time but is notable for Morrison's closed-lip vocal in the final chorus, and less so for the studio talk at the end as the band wonders whether or not it's a take.

The potential soul classic 'I've Been Working' might have been a good choice for a single but perhaps another woeful sax solo put the mockers on that. The high point of the song comes at the fade-out, as the band starts slipping fully into the groove, but the singles market has no time for such indulgence and it seems as though the best bit was left on the studio floor.

'Call Me Up in Dreamland' was a single, but its only credentials are really that it's as close as Morrison ever came to writing bubblegum music, while his over-singing of it — not unlike the soul-masters Pickett, Redding and Percy Sledge — creates a tension between what is said and how it's said. So too does the lyric, which pays homage to saxophones, while doing quite unspeakable things to one of them in yet another unfortunate solo. In common with a number of cuts on *His*

Nothing but a stranger in this world (1968–1974)

Band, 'Call Me Up in Dreamland' features the backing singing of the so-called Street Choir, one of whom was Janet Planet (whose duties also extended to waxing lyrical about Van's 'secret self' in the album's liner notes). The result is more enthusiastic than choral.

The highlight of the album comes on the reflective 'I'll Be Your Lover Too', with Morrison's vocals trading off against Platania's acoustic guitar and Shaar's brushes in a kind of Delta blues. It's part 'House of the Risin' Sun' and part Morrison's own trademark slow-burner, the mood tastelessly disrupted at the end by another snatch of studio talk. It's one of those unfortunate moments where the mystical mood-creator runs head first into the journeyman singer, and the reverie becomes lost in the dispassionate act of work.

'Blue Money' follows, beginning what used to be side two of the album. It isn't half the song of its predecessor, making a feature as it does of the nonsense 'do-do-you-do, n'-do-do-you-do'. But, presumably because its unremarkable twelve-bar riff has a kind of commercial appeal, it was chosen as a single, with modest sales results.

The weakest point of the album comes with the next trio of songs. 'Virgo Clowns' has jangling acoustic guitar, with Platania adding mandolin, and some unpleasant illustrative laughter at the end. 'Gypsy Queen' is another curiosity, beginning and ending with a tinkling music-box jingle missing only the spinning ballerina, and with Morrison recreating his 'Crazy Love' head voice to dubious effect. (Little wonder he would use it sparingly thereafter.) The song is West Coast pap, but 'Gypsy Queen' does contain one 'new' significant Morrisonism, in the phrase 'rave on'. In later years this would come to occupy a revered position in the singer's phrasebook, not just in the 1983 song 'Rave on, John Donne' but as an occasional visitor to live scats as well.

The formulaic, 'baby'-riddled twelve-bar blues of 'Sweet Jannie', which follows, also has little to commend it. More promising is 'If I Ever Needed Someone', in which the backing singers (unlike on 'Domino') repeat Morrison's lines and add some 'woo-ooh's of their own. It's arguably the first Morrison recording in which he casts out his Irish accent, and the echo of American voices come back to answer him. A pity then that, as with several other songs on the album, it peters out short of its full development.

Finally, 'Street Choir' offers the sort of commercial gospel vein that would re-emerge in more extended form in the late '70s on *Wavelength* and *Into the Music*. There are some ragged entries from singers and band alike on this track, but it really does provide Morrison with the opportunity for a state-of-the-union address: 'I just can't see you now,' he sings, in 'my New World crystal ball.' It's as if he is leaving someone behind (someone he says he can no longer 'free') as he emerges into his new American world. For an artist as individual and distinctive as Morrison, the formulaic, would-be hits of *His Band and the Street Choir* just don't work to form a convincing whole. Certainly, the album never became the commercial blockbuster it was intended to be. It's Van doing Wilson Pickett, rather than himself, and his attempt to become an American partially founders on the limited vision of the genre, which he, as a boy in Northern Ireland listening to the radio and collecting LPs, inherited second-hand. Too devoted to and maybe even too much in awe of the genre to transform

Nothing but a stranger in this world (1968–1974)

it, he imitates it, brilliantly, but ultimately in a way that's devoid of the spark that he'd already proved he possessed in music of his own. Tellingly perhaps, such a charge would never be levelled against those other explorers of American roots music, the Band (four-fifths of whom were Canadians) and the very English Rolling Stones.

Over the next thirty or more years he would go on to churn out plenty more of these homage recordings (explicitly, in the case of the albums from the mid to late nineties), with skill and sometimes devotion, but selling himself short on who he actually is as a musician. That desire to pay homage was his strength, and even became the subject of many of his songs, but as the mixed bag of *His Band and the Street Choir* demonstrates, sometimes it made him try to become something that he wasn't, constraining his talent within just one strand of a revered medium.

TUPELO HONEY

(November 1971)

- Wild Night ▪ (Straight To Your Heart) Like a Cannonball ▪ Old Old Woodstock ▪ Starting a New Life ▪ You're My Woman ▪ Tupelo Honey ▪ I Wanna Roo You (Scottish Derivative) ▪ When That Evening Sun Goes Down ▪ Moonshine Whiskey

During 1969 and 1970, Van Morrison's imaginative and physical journeys westward had been halted by the relative peace and tranquillity he'd achieved in Woodstock. But as the lyrics of 'Starting a New Life' would soon indicate ('We're gonna move / Way on down the line / Girl, we been standing in one place for too long a time'), pastoral bliss in upstate New York was a passing phase, a time when Morrison enjoyed domestic harmony, kindred musical spirits — both *his* band and *the* Band — living close by, and proximity to the nature that he worshipped in his songs.

The after-effects of the Woodstock Festival in August 1969, and more particularly the hugely successful film of the event released the following year, ensured that the sleepy hamlet had become a Mecca for hippies and other cultural tourists. No matter that the actual festival had occurred more than fifty miles away at a dairy farm near Bethel. Morrison was alarmed at this invasion of the curious, but his career was taking him ever further from New York state anyway. Simultaneously, the lease on his Woodstock house expired and — as unthinkable as it must have seemed to anyone listening to the recently released *His Band and the Street Choir* or reading its liner notes — his marriage hit a rocky patch, with Janet harbouring desires to return to her native West Coast. The result was that, by the time *Tupelo Honey* was being written, the singer's creative focus had shifted further west.

Morrison's closest friend in the Band, singer/pianist Richard Manuel, dubbed him 'the Belfast Cowboy' at this time (celebrated in their duet '4% Pantomime' on the Band's *Cahoots*). More than any of Van's other releases from the period, *Tupelo Honey* justified the nickname. It's an Ulsterman singing about America, resulting in an album that just stops short of explicitly revealing the singer's childhood fascination with the Wild West and Buffalo Bill. Cowboy, or

Nothing but a stranger in this world (1968–1974)

rather, country-and-western influence was rife in the US music scene by 1971, building on Dylan's *John Wesley Harding* album of January 1968. The Byrds' *Sweetheart of the Rodeo* and Dylan's next opus, *Nashville Skyline*, served as the blueprints for this new 'country-rock' genre; while the Band's eponymous second album, the Grateful Dead's *American Beauty*, aspects of Credence Clearwater Revival, Bread and Crosby Stills Nash & Young all set the path that would soon result in the Eagles breaking sales records for soft rock music delivered as if in Stetsons and ten-gallon hats.

Tupelo Honey was destined to become a problematic 'transitional' album in Morrison's career. Having been written largely on the Eastern seaboard, it was recorded on the West Coast, following Van and Janet's move to Marin County outside San Francisco in April 1971. Far from being developed as a coherent album, a number of the tracks were leftovers from earlier projects. Some, such as the execrable '(Straight to Your Heart) Like a Cannonball' and 'I Wanna Roo You', probably should have stayed where they were on the discard shelf.

With its emotional core torn between the American East and West coasts, then, and its references to Tupelo, the Deep South and Arkansas, it is in many ways Van Morrison's most 'American' album. The notorious cover art accentuates that Americanism, with Van as the Whitmanesque American settler leading the virginal-looking Janet on her white horse. It's a pioneer image, and the sepia tones of the back cover only reinforce the impression, Van and Janet posing awkwardly in period dress, a cross between nineteenth-century pilgrims and the humourless couple in Grant Wood's *American Gothic*.

A working man in his prime

Three years after *Astral Weeks* had looked home across the Atlantic, the pioneer family had established itself in this new land, and in the grand tradition, was heading west to settle in the land of plenty, where the wife had family connections.

But interestingly, just as Morrison was reinforcing his American credentials so explicitly, around the periphery of *Tupelo Honey* there emerged the occasional, incidental reference to the British Isles generally, not just Northern Ireland, but to Morrison's Scottish heritage. As Janet led her husband west across the prairies, Van began to replay his paternal links with Hibernian and Caledonian culture — that same culture that had turned out so many of the original American pioneers. There's the curious description of 'I Wanna Roo You' as a 'Scottish derivative', while the melody of the title track owes more to Irish folk song than to American r&b (although Clinton Heylin is not entirely correct when he says that the melody of 'Tupelo Honey' would be reused many years later for the Celtic 'Why Must I Always Explain?', from 1991's *Hymns to the Silence*). And 'Caledonia' was how he termed his Soul Orchestra, the exceptional band that began to take shape around the time of the album.

On arriving in the San Francisco area, Morrison is reported to have commented on how the scene there reminded him of his early years in Belfast. Still, there was little about the choice of session musicians for *Tupelo Honey* to remind him of even his recent past in New York. Only the presence of Jack Schroer, Gary Malabar and Connie Kay ensured any continuity from his previous three albums — although Platania, Labes and Shaar would all make the journey from the East Coast soon enough. (Indeed, they'd be performing with

Nothing but a stranger in this world (1968–1974)

Van by September, when a much-bootlegged live-in-the-studio performance at Pacific High Recording Studios took place.) Another break with recent tradition was the hiring of a co-producer, Warner's staffer Ted Templeman, to oversee the sessions. Joining this group at Wally Heider Recording and Columbia Studios were a number of musicians who would go on to back Morrison on later albums also: Ronnie Montrose (John Platania's temporary replacement on lead guitar), Rick Schlosser (sharing drum duties with Malabar and Kay), John McFee (pedal steel) and Mark Jordan (piano).

The result of their combined toil was an album that emanates from the American heartland but captures a major artist in a state of flux, both personal and musical. As he confronted these problems and — according to Templeman (at this stage, not really a fan of the singer's personality) — drank his way through the recording sessions, Morrison turned out an album that, despite its manifest weaknesses, still contains two classics and much else that can be regarded as typical Morrison.

The opening track and lead single, the r&b-infused 'Wild Night', is one of *Tupelo Honey*'s finest moments. The distinctive opening riff was apparently invented in the studio by guitarist Ronnie Montrose and it gives the song its urgency, not to mention a stylistic resemblance to 'Domino'. But while the riff and the genre might be American in origin, the lyrics are pure Belfast-era Morrison, with the female lover invited to walk out in the wet, windy streets and dance away the wild night in question. Never on any Van Morrison album has the weather played such a vital role as it does throughout *Tupelo Honey*, where almost every song is set outdoors in wind or rain, sunshine or snow. And as one would expect from a pioneer, everything is about journeying — usually on foot — through the weather, the destination alternately love, romance or the dance.

The 'world' of 'Wild Night' is not so far removed from the heroic backstreets whose imagery would propel Bruce Springsteen onto the covers of *Time* and *Newsweek* less than four years later. The girls are dressing up to go out, the boys are out in the street looking sharp, jukeboxes roar out 'just like thunder', and there's a sense of Edenic perfection (or in Morrison's terminology, 'completion') about the wild, hormone-drenched street-scene. As with the 'Madame George'-style send-offs, while Springsteen might have done it better and in more extended form, there is every reason to acknowledge that Van actually reached this thematic territory some years before the Boss. 'Wild Night' was 'Born to Run' — and later in Springsteen's career, 'Atlantic City' — in embryonic form. The pioneer depicted on the *Tupelo Honey* album cover didn't discover Wild West America per se. Rather, he was opening up a vision of the nation which would soon be seen most clearly from the viewpoint of Asbury Park, New Jersey.

'(Straight to Your Heart) Like a Cannonball' is another outdoors song, although on this occasion the protagonist is walking in his backyard while doing that familiar Morrison thing of waiting for the sun to shine. Or perhaps waiting for inspiration to hit, which it never really does in this song, whose clunky rhythm and forced jollity have 'filler' written all over them. Despite this, 'Like a Cannonball' was chosen as the album's third single (after 'Wild Night' and the title track), showing that, as with the songs selected for release off *His*

Nothing but a stranger in this world (1968–1974)

Band and the Street Choir, '45s' didn't necessarily constitute the best of their parent albums.

'Old Old Woodstock' is a homecoming song. Daddy's been out on the road and now his anticipation of returning to give his child 'a squeeze' is conceived in terms of the wind rushing around his coat and the cool night breeze blowing in his face. As so often in Morrison's music, it's a song about transportation, but in this case it's not entirely clear whether Daddy's returning home on foot ('swaggering over the ridge') or, as described later in the same verse, 'driving along in my old beat-up car'. 'Old Old Woodstock' is built on the tension between the protagonist as an artist who's 'bound to roam' and a parent returning home to expectant children and — in a vision of female subservience much favoured by both Morrison and Dylan — a woman waiting by the kitchen door.

On 'Starting a New Life', Van is edgy. It's spring and he's 'shovelling the snow away' while thinking about starting anew; but the singer has been working so hard that he has little to say except that it's time to be moving on. A perfunctory song that sounds like bad Robbie Robertson (and there was plenty of that around at this time, on the concurrently released *Cahoots*), it can be interpreted either as Morrison talking about leaving his partner behind, or at best making a half-hearted effort to convince himself that the move west with Janet is a good idea. Either way, with the benefit of hindsight and the knowledge that the marriage was breaking down, 'Starting a New Life' sounds unnervingly like it's actually ending an old relationship, with gruffness and a distinct lack of grace.

The pleading 'You're My Woman', which follows, seems desperate in its protestations of love, while the assertion that

A working man in his prime

the woman is his 'sunshine' while he is her 'guiding light' might alone have necessitated the publication of *The Female Eunuch* the following year. Somehow though, for all the interpolated 'Lord have mercy's and claims of his heart being 'for you', Morrison doesn't sound engaged in either the music or the naked emotion of the lyrics. Normally this wouldn't matter — Van has made an art of turning disinterest into transcendence — but in this case the song, with its blatantly silly 'really, really, really real's, just isn't strong enough to carry it off.

After what are perhaps the weakest four consecutive songs on any Van Morrison album, the following track is a revelation. 'Tupelo Honey' is one for the ages, a seven-minute vision of beauty. The gentle organ of the song's introduction might be borrowed from Procol Harum's 1967 hit 'A Whiter Shade of Pale' but in Morrison's song it quotes the opening line of a hymn which seeks forgiveness ('Dear Lord and Father of Mankind'), leading to a gorgeous melody that apparently accompanies a song of praise to Morrison's 'angel of the first degree'. Ebbing and flowing with natural ease, the emotion surging and then relenting, pausing for thought, then bursting with passion, 'Tupelo Honey' is uncomplicated — even facile — in the sentiments it expresses; but its sense of light and shade and its rhythmic suppleness make it a world unto itself, capable of radical reinterpretation with only the most minor of variations in inflection. With the tempo picking up imperceptibly in the middle section, it's among the handful of Morrison songs that most typify the spacious feel of his inspiration at its height.

For a comparatively straightforward love song, 'Tupelo Honey' nevertheless contains a rare (perhaps unintentional)

Nothing but a stranger in this world (1968–1974)

reference to political activism at the start of the second verse: 'You can't stop us on the road to freedom / You can't stop us 'cause our eyes can see'. When Morrison sings these lines prematurely, as he does on the live version from *A Night in San Francisco* after the earlier lyrics have been given insipid treatment by Brian Kennedy, the effect is electrifying. But Morrison is no Bob Dylan. Political protest is dropped as quickly as it arises, and we're back immediately in the world of angels and the sweet honey of the bee. Still even before this, the song has worked its magic, establishing itself as the first Morrison recording to capture the hypnotic, transcendental mood of *Astral Weeks* while possessing radio-friendly accessibility and broad commercial appeal (albeit at a greater length than the standard three minutes).

The album then lurches from the sublime to the ridiculous, with the irredeemable 'I Wanna Roo You'. There's snow outside and a further snowstorm's brewing, but with John McFee's pedal-steel guitar wailing and a forced-sounding middle eight, there's every reason to believe that the singer's doing exactly as he says in the song — going nowhere and with no plans.

In the context, the simple bar-room boogie of 'When That Evening Sun Goes Down' sounds far less pedestrian than it would have amid its natural company of r&b numbers from *His Band and the Street Choir*. Again there are plenty of clichés here, most of all in the lines 'Little girl, take me by my hand / I want you, understand / I wanna be your loving man', as well as a familiar Morrison motif in his offering to go for 'a stroll in the clear moonlight'. The clumsy writing continues with his stated wish to nibble the lover on her 'little ear'.

A working man in his prime

Much more interesting and in part convincing is the album's closing track, 'Moonshine Whiskey', whose rapid changes in mood and tempo, carolling gospel choir, references to railway and aeroplane travel, and calls to 'wait a minute' bear all the hallmarks of vintage Morrison. Unfortunately, lyrics such as 'Gonna put on my hot pants / And promenade down funky Broadway / 'Til the cows come home / La la la da . . .' and the reference to fish blowing bubbles render the song absurd just as it's approaching sublimity. Still, musically 'Moonshine Whiskey' demonstrates an epic vein of inspiration that the singer would wisely tap into again. The same multi-part structure would reach its initial climax in 'Listen to the Lion' (written at the same time but held over until the next album), before being used to more telling effect in Morrison's 'British' epics of the 1980s, such as 'Summertime in England' and 'In the Garden'.

On the evidence of *Tupelo Honey* as a whole, heading west had caused a shakedown in Morrison's art, revealing greatness and mortality in equal measure. Van himself has spoken of his dissatisfaction with the album, which never truly materialised as the country-and-western epic he'd imagined. Instead, it's a collection of songs that indicates a talented artist in unsettled mode, constantly attempting to reassure his loved one about their relationship while always looking for some way out. If nothing else, on the plus side it served to clear the way for the masterpiece of *Saint Dominic's Preview*, which was to emerge from California just nine months later.

The best and worst of Van Morrison that *Tupelo Honey* embodies would not only shape the Belfast Cowboy's future career, but that of many other major musicians too, including Springsteen in his greatest works, the young Elvis Costello (on

Nothing but a stranger in this world (1968–1974)

Almost Blue) and the mature Mark Knopfler (on *Sailing to Philadelphia*). Morrison the pioneer had explored America, but while he was doing so, he was simultaneously making plans to start a new life, and with his New World family collapsing, soon the Irishman's thoughts would turn homewards.

SAINT DOMINIC'S PREVIEW
(August 1972)

▪ *Jackie Wilson Said (I'm in Heaven When You Smile)* ▪ *Gypsy* ▪ *I Will Be There* ▪ *Listen to the Lion* ▪ *Saint Dominic's Preview* ▪ *Redwood Tree* ▪ *Almost Independence Day*

The further west Van Morrison travelled, the further east his thoughts seemed to turn. And the more Californian he became, the more British were his preoccupations and obsessions. Certainly, he was still working in the fields of American r&b and soul, and undoubtedly his American obsession endured, as it would for many decades thereafter. But as his marriage crumbled and his music reasserted itself as the dominant force in his life, he sought — unconsciously, no doubt, and within the context of simply 'working a job' — to redefine himself as a British artist.

By the time the magnificent *Saint Dominic's Preview* album was under way in early 1972, Morrison was busy establishing a 'Caledonian' empire in California. Although it wouldn't be used for this album, his new sixteen-track home recording studio in Fairfax, Marin County, bore the title 'Caledonia', just like his Soul Orchestra. And his production and publishing companies also bore the same title. Reticent to address his Belfast heritage at a time when his hometown was torn by sectarian violence (such matters were not an appropriate topic for a show-band performer), Morrison instead moved his imaginative identity further east, to the Scotland of his father's ancestry and the place of his earliest touring gigs abroad. This was the independent world north of Hadrian's Wall, where the Romans had never penetrated and where the fortress mentality and proud defiance of foreign culture had remained intact for centuries.

For the time being, and perhaps for evermore, Van Morrison became a proud Scot, relentlessly, obstinately and most of all rudely resisting overtures of appeasement and rapprochement from those marauding hordes who would claim his imaginative lands as their own. From that time on, those who wished to penetrate the Morrison defences first had to contend not just with the impregnable wall that had been constructed to keep them out, but also the abuse of the sentries manning the parapets. 'Caledonia' was an escape and a haven, and for one brief moment, in California, while he constructed its fortress walls, Van Morrison would turn out an album that encapsulated everything his extraordinary musical vision could imagine.

The first thing to be said about the wonderful *Saint Dominic's Preview* is that it is not rock 'n' roll. From the very opening phrases (scat-singing 'Do do do-do do / Do-do-do do do') to the last hypnotic bars of the wayward, mesmeric conclusion to 'Almost Independence Day', this is an album that drives the crooning of Tony Bennett and Frank Sinatra into mythical, mystical landscapes tinged with soul, jazz and folk. It

Nothing but a stranger in this world (1968–1974)

is, without doubt, the true follow-up to *Astral Weeks*, creating its own sound-world, its own genre, and most of all, its own sense of time and timelessness, as the uniformly strong songs set their own directions and agendas. No longer concerned with churning out potential hits, the Van Morrison who to some extent had been driven out of Woodstock to California, and who was now almost twenty-seven years old — the same age at which Hendrix, Joplin and Jim Morrison had all died — began to assert his own identity in a way that had not been possible since those New York sessions back in 1968.

Musicians of all types gathered for the recording, which took place at the same locations as the previous album, as well as Pacific High Recording Studio, also in San Francisco. On *Tupelo Honey* the drumming duties had been shared among three musicians, but on the new album, for the first time, there was no core band at all. Joining Van on guitar were three players, including Doug Messenger and Ronnie Montrose, whose contribution to *Tupelo Honey* had been one of its high points. Four drummer/percussionists appeared, including the previous trio of Gary Malabar, Rick Schlosser and Connie Kay; and there were two bassists. John McFee (on pedal steel) and Mark Jordan (piano) both made repeat appearances; while horn leader Jack Schroer finally found a partner in saxophonist Jules Broussard who would also be invited back again. The other keyboard players included Mark Naftalin, who had backed Van and John Lee Hooker on the latter's sessions in September '71 (the results of which would be heard on Hooker's 1972 album *Never Get Out of These Blues Alive* and the following year's *Born in Mississippi, Raised up in Tennessee*).

A working man in his prime

In short, under the guidance of co-producer Ted Templeman, there were jazz and blues and country musicians and even heavy rockers. The fruits of this union might easily have proved unfocused. But in one of those 'shazam!' moments of popular music — one thinks of Bob Marley taking on the Barrett brothers as a rhythm section — the right musical chemistry emerged and the different areas of musical specialisation somehow coalesced in a collection of songs that to this day defies genre and style. Even now, *Saint Dominic's Preview* could be described as the definitive Van Morrison album.

The scattish (but by no means skittish or Scottish) opening of the album sounds trite and out of tune for a moment before the hand claps and then Schroer's horns add to the energy. The band swings in and suddenly the music is jumping out of the speakers. There is a freshness and vitality in this opening number that has never been exceeded in Van Morrison's career. More particularly, it represents an explicit homage to the creator of 'Reet Petite', the great soul singer Jackie Wilson. Morrison's song title pointedly, and for the only time in his career, mentions the name-checked artist, with the more obvious title ('I'm in Heaven When You Smile') only appended as an afterthought.

On this song, Morrison presents one of his heroes in biblical terms, Jackie Wilson preaching the gospel of popular music and reiterating its stock phrases: 'let it all hang out', 'boom boom boom', augmented by Morrison's own 'ding-a-ling's. Years later Bruce Springsteen would, more explicitly, pronounce that he was 'preaching the ministry of rock 'n' roll', but he was only doing what Van Morrison had already

Nothing but a stranger in this world (1968–1974)

done (albeit in a non–rock 'n' roll context). 'Jackie Wilson Said' is the song — and *Saint Dominic's Preview* the album — that Bennett and Sinatra might have made had they been born into the postwar generation.

Imbued with the spirit and the gestures of mainstream pop, 'Jackie Wilson Said' remains one of Morrison's best singles. Though only a minor US hit at the time, it transcends time, place and genre while remaining true to its creator's show-band, brass-heavy roots. Populist though it may be, it's hard to imagine the song having been written or performed by anyone else — although Dexy's Midnight Runners would give it a try ten years later. It truly does swing.

The energy is sustained into the second track, bearing that already-familiar Morrison title of 'Gypsy'. Again the horns are to the fore, and in spite of its minor key, the song itself is a musical celebration, its rhythm and tempo variations seeming to tear itself apart, but all within the boundaries of its own form. It's a song about the desire to roam, with the moon above the gypsy-soul's head, and 'the road beneath your feet'. Drummer Rick Schlosser's brushed cymbals drive the music, pushing into one mood and then lurching back to another.

As in virtually all the tracks on this often 'wordless' album, Morrison makes plenty of use of 'la la la's and 'lie lie lie's. The ominous sound of the alternate section is contradicted somewhat by the singer's innocuous claims that camping beneath the stars 'can be so much fun'. 'Gypsy' survives its lyrical ineptitude, however, the rolling and swaggering feel of the opening returning us to the notion that wherever you lay your hat is your home ('check it out first' though, the singer cautions).

A working man in his prime

The crooner/lounge-jazz-singer side of Morrison's personality then emerges in 'I Will Be There', the closest number to a filler that this inspired album has. It's a big-band vein that the singer would return to throughout his career, although it's difficult to think of any highlights emanating from this particular strand of his musical personality. Again the horns are prominent, and there are plenty of indications that this was a performer who grew up working in show bands, but the song itself remains a confident and viable contribution to a working band's repertoire rather than the kind of ruminative act of contemplation that would typify this particular performer at his most original.

That quintessential, self-reflecting genius returns immediately though, in 'Listen to the Lion', a track that features on virtually everybody's list of major Van Morrison songs. 'The Lion' in question is intended to be Leo rising in Van's Virgo horoscope but in many ways the lyrics are irrelevant: they are mere vehicles on the journey to the heart and soul of Van Morrison's art.

The studio version is more to the point even if the live take on *It's Too Late to Stop Now* is perhaps the more penetrating of the two. But there is, and can be, no definitive version of 'Listen to the Lion' because the song is like a mantra, changing with the mood of the moment, its step-wise melodic and harmonic progression breathing with the ebb and flow of inspiration. Ostensibly it's a self-portrait — a depiction of the irascible genius whose violent outbursts are inspired by love and passion — but the tone now is more of sadness than anger.

The crucial word is 'listen', which throughout Morrison's career was to become a staple in live performance. Occurring regularly when the music comes down in volume (for instance, in 'And the Healing Has Begun' from 1979's *Into the Music*), it's another example of the artist's anti-rock 'n' roll stance. The moments in Van Morrison songs that are truly typical are always quiet. Indeed, musicians working with him at the time of *Saint Dominic's Preview* attest to his repeated assertion that he didn't want loud screaming guitars anywhere on his albums — and this at the time when Jimmy Page, Ritchie Blackmore and Eric Clapton reigned supreme in rock music. Here in 'Listen to the Lion', one gains the impression that, more than ever, the singer really does make a genuine effort to communicate with his listeners, in an act of self-revelation that he would subsequently abandon in favour of the whingeing 'Why Must I Always Explain?'. Given just how beautiful a song 'Listen to the Lion' is, one can understand his frustration that his self-portrait, obscure and enigmatic though it may be, can be universally praised on one hand but somehow ignored on the other.

In reality, the Van Morrison depicted in 'Listen to the Lion' is an apologetic bully, forgivable if only because he lacks hypocrisy and demonstrates at least some degree of self-knowledge. His gentle description of all his love coming 'tumbling down' is genuinely affecting, and his roaring pleas for the lion inside of him to be heard possess a degree of humanity that is uncharacteristic of much of his other work. When he promises to search his 'very soul' for the lion within him, it's a wonderfully human moment in which he simultaneously promises to understand himself better while also releasing his animal passion. (What woman could resist?) It becomes a song of repentance and of future promise.

Vocally, 'Listen to the Lion' is a tour de force, progressively moving from normal lyrics to all manner of vocalisations, from gruff grunts and unamused harrumphs through to a lion's roars, glottal stops, humming, quasi-coloratura flourishes, Sinatra 'da da da's and 'do do do's, bowel-straining sounds, some humming motor effects, a touch of keening and ranting, and smatterings of outright screaming and shouting — all of them distinctive examples of Morrison's speaking in tongues. There's something amazing inside this man, and over *Astral Weeks*-style accompaniment he lets it out with almost embarrassing candour and integrity.

And where does this most revelatory of Van Morrison songs end up? Sailing off via Denmark to Caledonia, that's where. It's as if the shattered would-be American is leaving his New World troubles behind and, for the second time in consecutive albums, is 'looking for a brand new start'. But now that object of the quest doesn't lie in the West. Whispering, almost as if it's a secret, childlike adventure, Morrison plans the route from San Francisco's Golden Gate way up to New York City.

Van Morrison's first seven solo albums pivot around this miraculous, groundbreaking meditation of a song, with its intellectual and thematic worlds reversing the westward trend and in fully considered form beginning his journey homeward — the journey that would result, with only one intervening album, in the climactic homecoming of *Veedon Fleece*. In this time capsule of a song, the by-now-familiar gypsy traveller, the immigrant, the stranger in a strange land, and most of all the lover of American music, begins to reassert his roots, psychologically, spiritually and philosophically. From this point,

Nothing but a stranger in this world (1968–1974)

the 'cry for home' will become an ever-increasing thematic preoccupation of his work. The elastic band that extended from Belfast to San Francisco reached its logical extension and the inevitable next action would be the slingshot effect propelling the artist home.

And that's why 'Listen to the Lion' represents a search for a centre. It's not just the lion inside Morrison that is being sought in the song; it's a search for identity itself, a quest for place and meaning and a source of belonging. Impressive enough on a purely musical level, it is also a triumph of the human spirit in the face of marital break-up. Refusing to bow to the typical self-doubt of the soon-to-be-divorced, the singer searches for the very sources of his strength and self-belief, beast-like though they might be. And while he yells and roars about it, he confronts his own vulnerability. So often the butt of listener's jokes, in 'Listen to the Lion', Morrison becomes more heroic than he would ever be again. For these reasons and much else besides, the song justifies its position at the pinnacle of his art.

But he's not done yet, because no sooner has 'Listen to the Lion' meandered off on its mythical journey back to Caledonia than Tom Salisbury's piano plays a few ballad-like introductory phrases to the title track. The instrumental opening of 'Saint Dominic's Preview' briefly lunges into the minor and sets its assured course straight into the heart of the singer's early life, with the first appearance of the window-cleaner image, later to become a familiar Morrison motif.

Apparently the St Dominic's church of the title had stuck in Morrison's mind, and only subsequently did he discover a newspaper reference to a peace service being held in just such a church in Northern Ireland. With Edith Piaf being name-checked, we are supposed to hear a blues version of 'Non Regredior' (presumably a misquotation of 'Non, je ne regrette rien'), but forget tragic French chanteuses; the first verse of the song places itself right at the centre of Morrison's world view: Northern Ireland, his teenage job (as a window cleaner) and popular music. Yet in spite of the excitement in the instrumental introduction — and there is no more urgent opening to any Van Morrison song — the narrator still remains firmly in San Francisco 'trying hard to make this whole thing blend'.

'Saint Dominic's Preview' is the theory of 'Listen to the Lion' put into practice, with the cultural clash between America and the British homeland exacerbated by geographical distance. No one is home. Drummer Gary Malabar (as he later admitted in describing the song's origins) is missing his lifestyle away across the continent in upstate New York, while Van is thinking about his own home, hence the untypically self-revealing lines 'And it's a long way to Buffalo / It's a long way to Belfast City too'. The homesickness that would one day result in an album of Irish folk songs with the Chieftains reveals itself in rare and explicit form in this song.

An impartial listener might conclude that California was freaking Morrison out. In response, the visions that he was having of Northern Ireland were but a 'preview' of what was to come; the man needed to get back home, hire a car, and go and see some of his own country. But that would still be a year or more away. Meanwhile, the miseries and delusions of the American dream — supermarket dwellers not feeling 'anyone

Nothing but a stranger in this world (1968–1974)

else's pain' or making commitments 'to anybody but themselves' — were still fuelling this classic Morrison song, with his American backing musicians in exceptional form, pushing on with the closest brush with social protest that Morrison would ever achieve.

He sees the vision of Hank Williams's America, with its 'chains, badges, flags and emblems', but his real gaze is now towards the land of St Dominic and the other Irish saints. Right here, it's just record company schmoozing and socialising, trying to 'be hip and get wet with the jet set'. The singer keeps his eye on the return home, but this final stanza also points the way forward (if 'forward' is the correct word) to that unfortunate slew of songs, typified by the near-contemporary 'Drumshambo Hustle' and the subsequent 'Big Time Operators', slagging off the music business. In its infancy, however, the images of hypocrites and cheats in the American record industry are merely distractions from the inspired view homeward, not the very substance of the ungracious and pedestrian songs that they would later become. 'Saint Dominic's Preview' spits bile on a creative level akin to Dylan's 'Positively 4th Street' and John Lennon's 'How Do You Sleep?', because it is conveyed within the context of a broader, inspirational vision.

Meanwhile, in among these profound thoughts of adulthood, the childlike vision once more comes creeping into view, with a boy and his dog walking by the river and across the fields — 'looking for the rainbow', 'laughing all the way' — in the joyously naive 'Redwood Tree'. The sheltering tree in question is the only thing about the song that's American, for the remainder is a classic Morrison ballad of childhood, complete with the boy and his father searching for the lost dog, and the inevitable rain and impending thunder. A perfect choice for the album's second single, surprisingly it failed to make any impression when released in late 1972. (The same fate befell 'Gypsy', the third single.)

'Redwood Tree' is a Blakean song of innocence replete with a deceptively grim introduction leading to a buoyant tune, and speculations about thunder as a dark premonition in an otherwise perfect natural landscape. Sandwiched between two epics on side two of the original LP, 'Redwood Tree' has always been underrated, but there are few other Morrison songs that capture so perfectly his take on the contrast between innocence and experience. More than a decade before the appearance of *A Sense of Wonder*, 'Redwood Tree' surely indicates the singer's familiarity with the work of William Blake much earlier than is usually acknowledged.

Straightaway though, we're back into the world of keening at the opening of the pointedly titled 'Almost Independence Day'. The vocals trading off against slide guitar pre-empt the work of Harry Manx in their blending of oriental and blues scales. They merge into more predictable harmonies as the band kicks in — introducing the Moog synthesizer for the first time in his career — and Van is with his lady in Chinatown, hearing echoes all the way from Oregon.

Thematically, the album's sequence makes no sense. At one level, this song set on the shores of San Francisco Bay in the (usual) 'cool, cool night' still has Morrison lodged firmly in America, as if 'Listen to the Lion' had never happened. But then contradicting an impression was always Morrison's way, turning an album that clearly points the way homeward into

Nothing but a stranger in this world (1968–1974)

just another collection of songs. As he looks out there on the harbour, he's pointing the way forward (almost note-perfectly) to his 1991 collaboration with John Lee Hooker on 'I Cover the Waterfront'.

And yet there remains a disconcerting ambiguity. Of course on a literal level, it's almost the American national holiday, the Fourth of July, but the imagery is more complicated than that. The fireworks are bursting 'up and down the San Francisco Bay', but Morrison's eyes are fixed on the harbour; and the song, far from arousing patriotic feelings about 'the land of the free', inhabits that epic, meditative space this singer always employs for his most deeply personal utterances. In fact, Morrison is taking the United States' celebration of national identity and turning it into a symbol of his own escape and of the search for his own, Caledonian identity. (Bruce Springsteen would do something very similar in his 1980 song 'Independence Day', and so would Richard Ford in his 1995 novel of the same name.) Morrison wants independence *from* America, and from Janet and the record industry. He wants out, and as he gazes at the harbour, he knows it's almost *his* independence day.

Paradoxically, given that this was the first album since *Astral Weeks* where Morrison seemed unconcerned with commercial success, *Saint Dominic's Preview* peaked higher on the US album charts (at number 15) than any of his previous releases. Although Morrison's albums are no strangers to the British Top 10, this remains his highest-charting album in America. And, for the first time since *Moondance* two-and-a-half years before, the critics were lauding his new record.

A working man in his prime

It was the right album at the right time, capturing the mood of the moment. By turns uplifting and homesick, optimistic but wary, and most of all irresistibly sung, played and written, it remains one of the great works in the Morrison canon. The sense of longing, exile and looming fatigue that pervades *Saint Dominic's Preview* was something that most survivors of the 1960s could share. It was as close as Morrison would ever come to expressing the voice and the conscience of his generation.

HARD NOSE THE HIGHWAY
(July 1973)

■ *Snow in San Anselmo* ■ *Warm Love* ■ *Hard Nose the Highway* ■ *Wild Children* ■ *The Great Deception* ■ *Bein' Green* ■ *Autumn Song* ■ *Purple Heather*

By 1973 popular music had begun to take itself very seriously indeed, aligning its style with the great classics and in many cases actually incorporating choirs, orchestras and other trappings of symphonic form into music of mass appeal. Deep Purple, the Moody Blues and Procol Harum had long since made recordings with symphony orchestras; Pink Floyd were turning out albums consisting of songs that lasted an entire side of an LP; and artists such as Jethro Tull were actually going the whole way with single-number albums. Meanwhile, Emerson Lake and Palmer were showing off their classical training, Yes were at the vanguard of progressive rock's orchestral fixation, and the arrival of the Moog synthesizer meant that pop music could achieve a massed orchestral

Nothing but a stranger in this world (1968–1974)

sound at the push of a button. Most of all, rock operas like *Tommy* and *Jesus Christ Superstar* were the talk of the music industry.

Into this world of vaulting musical ambition and self-important excess staggered an exhausted Van Morrison, who in the space of some two-and-a-half years had turned out four albums of original material. And now, so soon after completion of the masterly *Saint Dominic's Preview*, terminally separated from his wife and child, touring extensively with the Caledonia Soul Orchestra — including a series of gigs at LA's Troubadour club, one of which would make up much of his live set released the following year — and with the world of music changing all around him, he had to do it all again. By early 1973, the weary Ulsterman was putting together a new album to build on the commercial success that he was at last beginning to achieve.

While his heroes remained r&b and soul artists, Van himself wasn't immune to classical influence. At this time the Soul Orchestra included a small string section which interspersed the nightly set with smatterings of classical music, including Vaughan Williams's *The Lark Ascending*. But the fundamentally improvisatory nature of Morrison's music made it less suitable for 'classical' adaptation than that of many of his contemporaries.

Nevertheless, what emerged out of this chaotic time was *Hard Nose the Highway*, an album that began smack-bang in the world of opera, and ended with an entire LP side consisting of over-long and unconvincing lounge jazz. The songs' landscapes were almost entirely those of autumn and winter, with moments of inspiration offset by whinges about the fickleness and opportunism of the professional music industry.

A working man in his prime

Rob Springett's cover painting serves as a warning: Van, it seems, has turned his back on the horrors of modern urban life and instead crouches peacefully, surveying the firmament. Beneath a starry sky are green fields, blue cows, a human figure struggling to disentangle itself from a bed sheet, and an elderly Oriental man who might or might not be Ho Chi Minh. In an interview recorded shortly after the album's release, Morrison revealed that the cover imagery had come out of a long discussion he had had with the artist. When Van saw the finished artwork it apparently accorded with his mental state. 'That's exactly what I'm thinking,' he told Donal Corvin.

Recorded at Morrison's home studio in Fairfax, the sessions brought together all of the official Caledonia Soul Orchestra line-up (bar the drummer, Dahaud Shaar). John Platania and Jeff Labes both made vinyl contributions for the first time since 1970, then, while other members of the live band — bassist David Hayes, trumpeter Bill Atwood and the string players led by violinist Nathan Rubin — were making their first appearance on a Van Morrison album. Studio regulars Jack Schroer (the one constant in the live and studio line-ups from 1970 to 1974), Gary Malabar and Rick Schlosser also featured. Sharing the production credits with the singer this time around were Labes and Schroer, rather than record-company stooge Ted Templeman, whose presence, one imagines, would hardly have been conducive to the anti-industry sentiments of much of the material.

Whether or not a disciplined (and disciplinarian) co-producer would have made a difference, the resulting album was a mess, yet it has its moments. Thematically, it is all about

Nothing but a stranger in this world (1968–1974)

fatigue: being tired of the road, tired of the business, tired of all the charlatans and tired of, in Morrison's own words, 'the great deception'. After the uplifting, inspired nature of its predecessor, *Hard Nose the Highway* is one of the biggest downers of this natural pessimist's career.

It begins like no other Morrison album. A celestial choir (in fact, the Oakland Symphony Orchestra's chamber chorus) sings what sounds like, but isn't, something from Vaughan Williams's *Shepherds of the Delectable Mountains*. One can imagine the shock of a listener expecting the catchy r&b and soul riffs that had opened the previous three albums but suddenly hearing a heavenly choir intoning a weather report that it's snowing somewhere in northern California. It's an ambitious task, marrying the soulful vocals of a rock singer with the stentorian, four-square approach of the choir (something that Pink Floyd had done rather better with the John Aldiss Choir's contribution to *Atom Heart Mother* three years before), but the variations of rhythm and tempo almost create enough diversity to bring it off.

More particularly, the sound of 'Snow in San Anselmo', with its choral effects and galloping bass underneath, bears a striking resemblance to Uriah Heep's epic *Salisbury* album, released in 1971. One of the great cult classics of the so-called 'prog-rock' phenomenon — and Uriah Heep's only sustained venture into the genre — it's hard to imagine that Morrison was unfamiliar with it when cutting 'Snow in San Anselmo'. The use of Moog synthesizer in 'Almost Independence Day' notwithstanding, this opening track of *Hard Nose the Highway* would be a rare foray for this purist white soul singer into the inflated world of art-rock.

A working man in his prime

The event being described was in fact the first such snowfall in the area in thirty years. Morrison, in town that February for a gig at the Lion's Share (and later for a recording session at the Church studio with Ronnie Montrose and others), weaves around it an impressionistic portrait of the district — the mission in San Rafael, the massage parlour and the 24-hour pancake house among them. Symbolically, the fact that snow is falling in California is not without significance, for the circumstances of Morrison's life are surely encapsulated in the meteorological metaphor. He was successful, admired and had a flourishing career, but personal trauma and fatigue — like freakish weather — obey no rational laws, and this strange album would begin the culture of complaint that subsequently came to typify the most ill-tempered moments of the singer's future career.

In this particular track though, the curiosity value sustains the listener's interest in what is undoubtedly the most 'classical-sounding' song that Morrison has ever recorded. As in so many of Morrison's narrative set-ups, the radio is playing, but this time it's not r&b from Radio Luxembourg but 'the classic music station'; and, unlike in 'Caravan', it's not being turned up with menace, but instead 'plays in the background soft and low'. There's silence around the cascades as the singer prepares for the beginning of an opera, which according to the ridiculously dramatic choir seems to 'suddenly appear'. To accommodate the expanded (quasi-symphonic) musical horizons of the piece, Morrison employs clashing vocal registers, the head voice suddenly being answered with chest notes, and vice versa. Clearly it's an experiment, and while it's a genre that he would never explore

Nothing but a stranger in this world (1968–1974)

further, it does raise expectations for the creative direction of the album that follows.

The second track, though, returns immediately to more familiar territory, with 'Warm Love' being a rather too-similar replay of 'Crazy Love' from *Moondance*, complete with the same head voice. The accompaniment includes an equally timid flute, as well as backing vocals by Jackie DeShannon, for whom Van would write and produce four songs around this time (only one of which, 'Sweet Sixteen', would get an immediate release). It's the usual scenario of Morrison's love songs: the destination is the country in sunshine, and when evening comes on a few campfire-style songs accompanied by guitar, but then it starts raining and the lovers leave for their warm hearth where they can dry out their clothes. Unexceptional, although typical, in every way, 'Warm Love' could have fitted anywhere on *Moondance*, *His Band and the Street Choir* or *Tupelo Honey*, a fact no doubt that made it the logical choice for the album's first single.

More interesting is the title track, a song so personal and self-revelatory that it might have been an out-take from *Saint Dominic's Preview*. In another emphatically anti-rock 'n' roll gesture, Morrison name-checks Frank Sinatra and the string section of Nelson Riddle's orchestra as models for his own professional studio technique, where he (to this day) likes to blow in and out and then 'takes a vacation'. In the chorus of 'Hard Nose the Highway' he complains that he's seen 'hard times', drawn 'fine lines' and hasn't had 'time for shoe shines', but naturally this all resolves into the classic Morrison ploy of hitting the road again — hence the title of the song.

A working man in his prime

The second verse alludes momentarily to depression and difficult times in Boston and Belfast; while the final verse instructs music-industry executives (one imagines) to 'put your money where your mouth is', that is, take a gamble on an artist whose personality and spontaneous studio technique don't quite fit the mould. In declaring that 'in order to win you must be prepared to lose sometime', Morrison makes a moot point which summarises his whole career. The many bad performances and the slew of dreadful songs are more than compensated for by those moments when Van the Man is on song. Sadly, in this most self-aware of numbers, he is not, and the music to which the revealing lyrics are set is pedestrian and devoid of much interest.

The same is true of the next track, 'Wild Children', which is a curious slice of autobiography and the first of Morrison's extended name-check numbers. Essentially the song is a list of the popular-culture idols for those born, like Morrison himself, in 1945 — 'when all the soldiers came marching home'. 'We were the war children,' he sings in the first line (in the live version on *It's Too Late to Stop Now*, however, it's 'wild children' all the way through the song). The idols turn out to be a fairly predictable list of American method actors, James Dean taking his 'fatal ride', Rod Steiger and Marlon Brando together in some half-remembered image from *On the Waterfront*. More surprisingly, playwright Tennessee Williams gets a mention, as Van implores him to let his 'inspiration flow', and later, for some reason, to let it 'go'. Also flowing are the 'springtime rivers', and the music, with its gentle strumming and frankly informal approach to melody, never settles either. Like those springtime rivers, the backing on 'Wild Children' is meandering and hook-free.

Nothing but a stranger in this world (1968–1974)

Nevertheless, the sympathetic listener who has taken the previous track to heart will acknowledge that in order to win you have to be prepared to lose sometime, and so we press on. For that we are generously rewarded with 'The Great Deception', the wonderful song that closes what was side one on the original LP. With a strong melody and the most confident vocal on the album (apparently recorded with Morrison lying on his back while extemporising some of the lyrics), it's perhaps the definitive Van Morrison whinge song, its target being the 'world of lies' in which the singer lives.

'The Great Deception' begins with a jibe at 'plastic revolutionaries' who 'take the money and run', and from these hypocrites moves on through other smiling thieves to the 'self-righteous' who 'pin you up against the wall'. Vain rock 'n' roll singers also come in for a spanking, for their calls of 'power to the people' while owning 'three or four Cadillacs'. By contrast, we're asked if we've heard about 'the great Rembrandt' (as years later we'll be asked if we've heard 'about Wordsworth and Coleridge, baby'), who was so under-appreciated during his lifetime that he didn't even have money for his brushes. With bile being spat in all directions, it's as if Morrison is straining to achieve the venom of Bob Dylan at his most sarcastic, and by the time we've been through the Hollywood actor who ends up drunk and wasted in the Bowery, we arrive at the 'so-called hippies' who steal your eyeballs and then ask, 'Son, kid, do you want your eyeballs back?'. No doubt somewhere in the Morrison subconscious (as biographer John Collis points out), these latter lines recalled Dylan's snarling 'Ballad of a Thin Man', where Mr Jones's throat is returned with 'thanks for the loan'.

A working man in his prime

The second half of *Hard Nose the Highway* is all downhill from here, with three interminable tracks that sound like a cross between Frank Sinatra and Wilson Pickett singing mediocre lounge jazz. The descent into ignominy begins with the first non-Van Morrison original released during the artist's solo career. Wisely ignored by record buyers when issued as a single, it's a predictably eccentric choice in the Kermit the Frog song 'Bein' Green', written by Joe Raposo. Crying out perhaps for Morrison's Kermit-like head voice, 'Bein' Green' doesn't receive it, or any kind of inspiration for that matter, other than a half-baked Tony Bennett impersonation.

Still, the man is working, singing a song that people know well and might appreciate late at night in a bar, where they don't have to pay money for it and aren't too choosy about what they hear. Clearly at this point — where for the first time he held sole decision-making power over what went onto the album — Morrison didn't really value his status as the creator of masterpieces like *Astral Weeks* and *Saint Dominic's Preview*. He was a singer for hire. Buyer beware.

'Autumn Song', the only original of the final three tracks, is a jazzy little crooner's number with all the usual images: falling rain, the seasons, lovers walking around, putting coal on the fire, and chestnuts roasting on a crisp night. There is often music in Morrison's outdoors settings, of course, and on this occasion it's not the usual radio or campfire guitars but an 'old accordion man'. Apart from its comparatively sophisticated jazz-guitar chords, the only really noteworthy feature of this aimless piece is the improvisatory phrases at the end of the song. Like so much else on this strange album, in

Nothing but a stranger in this world (1968–1974)

'Autumn Song' there's the feeling of marking time, working a routine job and awaiting inspiration.

The first and only indication that something might be brewing, namely a return to form in the ensuing *Veedon Fleece*, comes in the album's final number. The Scottish traditional song 'Purple Heather' (sometimes known as 'Wild Mountain Thyme') was Morrison's first commercially released recording of a 'Caledonian' tune, and for a moment it seems as though the promise of *Saint Dominic's Preview* is to be fulfilled. Is this, at last, independence day? The answer is at best equivocal: yes, the song might be 'Caledonian', but the treatment is hardly that. On the contrary, 'Purple Heather' sounds no different from the songs that had preceded it on *Hard Nose the Highway*. It's lightweight and middle of the road, the road in question being Main Street, USA. Even the lyrics, with the opening reference to the changing of the seasons, might have been written by Morrison himself.

Two years previously, Van had delivered a mostly directionless album that served to clear the way for the masterpiece that was soon to follow in *Saint Dominic's Preview*. Similarly, if *Hard Nose the Highway* only delayed delivery of what 'Almost Independence Day' had promised, the next album would make amends. For now though, Morrison was facing his first widespread critical lambasting — even *His Band* and *Tupelo Honey* had received some very positive reviews. Yet while the songwriting on *Hard Nose the Highway* was below par, Morrison's live performances were electrifying around this time resulting in the creation of *It's Too Late To Stop Now*, recorded between May and July 1973, and rarely, if ever, bettered in terms of Morrison's live performance standards.

A working man in his prime

Creatively, however, it seemed Morrison was drawing breath for a new, and highly significant stylistic development. His gaze now firmly fixed on his homeland, he was ready to search for his roots in the green fields of Ireland. The failure of his sixth solo album would make the wonder of the successful seventh all the more impressive.

VEEDON FLEECE
(October 1974)

■ *Fair Play* ■ *Linden Arden Stole the Highlights* ■ *Who Was That Masked Man?* ■ *Streets of Arklow* ■ *You Don't Pull No Punches, But You Don't Push the River* ■ *Bulbs* ■ *Cul de Sac* ■ *Comfort You* ■ *Come Here My Love* ■ *Country Fair*

Although Van Morrison was probably oblivious to it during their conception, his first five studio albums chart a consistent course westwards until, on the final track of *Saint Dominic's Preview*, the singer looks back across the American continent and the Atlantic Ocean to focus on the place where he was born and raised. As once the Belfast youth had dreamed of America, on *Veedon Fleece* the American singer imagines Northern Ireland.

Yet Morrison himself could tell quite a different story, of how between those years 1972 and 1974 he had settled so comfortably into Californian life that he'd moved his parents away from the Troubles and set them up in a record shop of their own (naturally named 'Caledonia') near his home in Fairfax. He could point out that he was still so imbued with American culture that he was planning a country-and-western

Nothing but a stranger in this world (1968–1974)

album, after the disappointment of *Tupelo Honey*. And most of all, he could remind us — and indeed on several occasions he has — that each of the seven studio albums between 1968 and 1974 could have contained vastly different music from the material with which his fans are so familiar.

On this last score, there would certainly be some strength in his argument. The years 1973–74, in particular, saw Morrison record a huge number of songs that went unreleased at the time, judging by the track listing of *The Philosopher's Stone*. In 1973, for instance, as well as a session in San Anselmo with Ronnie Montrose (which produced the original version of 'Wonderful Remark'), Van recorded with Jackie DeShannon; and even after accounting for his own release, *Hard Nose the Highway*, there were still tracks left over from that album's sessions (including 'Drumshanbo Hustle', of course). The following year would see him producing an album of new material, as usual, and taking part in recording sessions at Hilversum's Wisseloord Studios, in Holland.

This period would also be one of his busiest in terms of touring. Aside from his gruelling schedule in 1973, in the first seven months of 1974 he toured America's Eastern seaboard, played in Europe (including at the prestigious Montreux Jazz Festival) and performed locally on the West Coast. If nothing else, in the middle of all this work and no play, the recently divorced Morrison needed a holiday.

Veedon Fleece was written in an inspired few weeks in October–November 1973, after the singer set foot in his native Northern Ireland for the first time in six years, accompanied by his new partner Carol Guida. While he didn't actually visit his strife-torn home city, the trip — from Dublin up to Ulster, and then back down south through Ireland — seemed to be just the tonic he needed. When he returned to America, Morrison was back in top form. The visit certainly appears to have had a profound effect on his music, with 'Astral Weeks', 'Ballerina' and 'Madame George' appearing prominently in the set lists for his US concerts the following February and March. And tellingly, this album's 'Streets of Arklow' would also be performed regularly, six months or more before its official release.

Returning to Caledonia Studios, the album sessions began in November 1973. By this stage, his Soul Orchestra had morphed into the Caledonia Soul Express, the result of which was that, of those who had appeared on the recently released *It's Too Late to Stop Now*, only Jack Schroer, Jeff Labes, David Hayes, Dahaud Shaar and two members of the string section, violinist Nathan Rubin and cellist Terry Adams, would join Van in the studio. Among the many one-off contributors this time around was session guitarist John Tropea.

One of his most cleverly written and truly innovative albums, *Veedon Fleece* brings together all the strains of his musical personality, consisting of songs that blend American gestures and themes with traditional Irish music in a manner that would influence a subsequent generation of Celtic folk-rockers. As personal and self-revelatory in its own way as *Saint Dominic's Preview*, for Van Morrison purists, *Veedon Fleece* holds a special place in the canon, as the work that most neatly and with considerable beauty summarises the artist's biography.

This synthesis begins right at the start, in the extraordinary two-chord waltz 'Fair Play'. Immediately, the

Nothing but a stranger in this world (1968–1974)

new Irish setting (so different in geographic location from all previous opening tracks since *Astral Weeks*) is made clear. We are in Killarney, deep in the south-west of Eire, with its blue lakes and 'architecture . . . so fine'. Wandering through the meadows of his native land, Morrison is thinking about Edgar Allan Poe, Oscar Wilde and Henry David Thoreau, but most surprisingly of all, given his recent albums, he's feeling 'love of life'. It's a positive mood that's sustained throughout the album as a whole, setting up, among much else, a set of love songs that are more giving and open in their emotion than any recorded before or since. 'Fair Play' is a kind of embryonic 'On Hyndford Street' (the centrepiece of his 1991 album *Hymns to the Silence*), wherein the encounter with the Irish landscape of Morrison's childhood, plus a paperback book, inspire 'tales of mystery . . . and imagination'. The Irish meadow is the source of dreaming but, crucially, and in what becomes a synthesis of all Morrison's juvenile influences, it's juxtaposed with cries of 'Geronimo' and 'hi ho, Silver', phrases remembered from cowboy serials in the Saturday morning cinema matinees of Morrison's childhood. Here at last — after six previous albums of cultural redefinition — the dual sources of the artist's formative inspiration are brought together. The Irish landscape and the popular culture of America pour through his mind with equal power as he walks down the Irish street with his sweetheart. After six years of expatriation, Van the Man was at last making sense of his cultural roots and offering acceptance, borrowing from Paul McCartney the heartfelt phrase 'Let it be'. Settle in for the ride. Van Morrison is taking us back with him — taking us way, way back.

A working man in his prime

'Linden Arden Stole the Highlights' vies for the award of Van Morrison's most obscure title but the song itself is another example of an inspired fusion between Irish and Wild West influence. The Linden Arden in question is a San Franciscan outlaw driven through his fondness for a drink to commit violence and become a gunslinger living in fear of his life. But the piano-ballad 'sound' of the song, with its beautiful, wide-ranging melody and subtle, supple rhythm (bars of two and four beats alternating regularly) is Irish. Like 'Fair Play', it offers evidence that Morrison's return to his homeland inspired Irish-sounding music but Wild West imaginings.

'Who Was That Masked Man?' (its title taken from *The Lone Ranger* television series) picks up on the final lines of 'Linden Arden' and depicts the fugitive hiding out, unable to trust anyone and as fragile as a butterfly 'all encased in glass'. A comparatively articulate song about being haunted and in fear of what's about to barge in through the door, it makes a curiously affecting self-portrait of Morrison himself, particularly given his later obsession with privacy. The song concludes with the observation that 'there's good and evil in everyone'. With his voice set high up in that distinctive, falsetto range, the normally bellowing, bellicose preacher-man actually sounds vulnerable. Like its two predecessors on the album, 'Who Was That Masked Man?' ends without a musical clincher, as if the sentiment from one song is meant to merge seamlessly into the next number, having drawn no conclusions and leaving the specific emotion up in the air.

But then in a rare masterstroke of track sequencing, these American dreams descend suddenly from a vague, floating G minor into an emphatic E minor and we're in the slow,

Nothing but a stranger in this world (1968–1974)

brooding world of 'Streets of Arklow' — its subject, its music, its entire demeanour grounded in the 'drenching beauty' of being back in Ireland. From the opening track's setting of Killarney, and the Wild West imagery in between, we're now transported to County Wicklow, on the country's east coast. The national identity depicted in this most ecstatic of songs is classified as a head filled with poetry, a gypsy's love of wandering (for Van Morrison the terms 'gypsy' and 'Irishman' seem almost synonymous), shining eyes and clean souls. That's what it means for Morrison to be Irish. And that's why his most uplifting songs are always set in Irish — or at least British — landscapes. America is where the work gets done, but as *Veedon Fleece* demonstrates so emphatically, it's in Ireland that the soul and the spirit are rejuvenated.

A recorder (doing the work of a tin whistle) sounds the counter-melody throughout 'Streets of Arklow', and it not only presages the subsequent collaboration with the Chieftains but also announces the homecoming of an Irish soul singer for whom no amount of Wilson Pickett or Sam Cooke impersonations can disguise musical roots laid firmly in the land where the green grass grows. As in 'Fair Play', these profound feelings of homecoming are captured in 'Streets of Arklow' through the employment of just two repeated chords, E minor and C major. It is as though the music itself is hammering home the simple truth that Van has returned to his roots.

The two chords don't change even when, in another smooth transition, the tempo steps up for the stupidly titled 'You Don't Pull No Punches, But You Don't Push the River' (perhaps Morrison was thinking about Joe Walsh's *The Smoker You Get, the Player You Drink*, released the year before). This extraordinary, extended meditation is Morrison in Philip Glass mode, the accompaniment in 12/8 time repeating endlessly while Morrison's 'da da da' vocal begins off-beat like a man dangerously clambering aboard a moving freight train. Once settled in, the ride goes a long way and in magnificent, noble style, out into the country and then on to the west coast (but this time of Ireland, of course), where the singer and his lover encounter the days of 'blooming wonder'.

The landscape encountered along the way is a mythical one peopled by William Blake and his Eternals, as well as the Sisters of Mercy, who are searching for 'the Veedon Fleece'. In Blake's epic poetry, the Eternals are immortals whose perceptions are extended beyond the range of normal human experience owing to their liberation from the confines of physical mortality. But in a surprisingly powerful poetic image, they, just like the Sisters of Mercy — the order of Catholic nuns made famous by Leonard Cohen in his song of that title — are all in search of the same mythical grail. It's a line that encapsulates many of the preoccupations that sustain Morrison's art, while the mention of the Eternals suggests that the songwriter's acquaintance with William Blake was more than fleeting.

Presumably the Veedon Fleece itself is Morrison's version of the Golden Fleece sought by Jason and the Argonauts. The object of the quest, however, is not as important as the search. Filled with wonder, Van is off with the poets and the preachers looking for spiritual enlightenment.

The names of these searcher-colleagues become a mantra for the meditation that 'You Don't Pull No Punches' essentially is. With that same two-chord pattern repeated over and over, eventually the song reaches a point of repose, even as Jim

Nothing but a stranger in this world (1968–1974)

Rothermel's blue-in-the-face flute line plays on; but it soon picks up again with the telling final verse, in which Indian guru Meher Baba gets to join the other searchers. Finally, the song winds down, as if the travellers are descending to the beach at sunset to begin some holy ceremony. An underrated gem in Morrison's oeuvre and a minimalist marvel composed in the same year as Glass's *Einstein On the Beach*, there is much in the music, lyrics and overall feel of 'You Don't Pull No Punches' to qualify it as one of the definitive achievements of the artist's career.

In a transition from deep spiritual ecstasy to the prosaic here and now, we're suddenly thrust into what appears to be the kick-off for a football game at the start of 'Bulbs', the album's hit single, and another track that had already been performed lived (at Montreux, in late June). Whoever it is that he's 'kicking off from centre field' to — and it's certainly not Blake and the Sisters of Mercy — they are soon replaced by a lover 'standing in the shadows' who is 'leaving for an American'. Apparently 'her batteries are corroded' and 'her hundred-watt bulb just blew', but somehow those clues don't seem to help very much in deciphering this upbeat, engaging song whose most illuminating lyrics are the guttural 'la la la's of the chorus. Halfway through we hear that her brothers and sisters are standing 'on Atlantic sand', presumably not with her in the shadows, then, 'where the street lights all turn blue'. But with the tune's boppy mood, it doesn't seem to matter because, as the song itself says in a fleeting moment of coherence, 'it's all showbiz'. And if nothing else, 'Bulbs' moves a step away (to C major and four chords) from the thirteen-minute cycle of E minor/C major chord changes that preceded it.

A working man in his prime

Much more revealing lyrically — and quite intriguing musically, if only for its grunting vocals at the end, which sound like a warthog feeding — is 'Cul de Sac', a glorious and explicit celebration of homecoming. Recounted from a familiar 'hideaway', Morrison confesses that 'it's been much too long since we drifted in song' from that wet place. It's a song about travelling long distances, meeting lots of people, but when they go home, the singer himself will 'double back' to his own private cul-de-sac, a point of origin that can only be left, not travelled beyond.

The mere thought of it transforms Morrison into a keening Irishman, 'Cul de Sac' moving beyond words into a visceral embodiment of the most private, intimate and non-commercial of folk vocalisations. Morrison couldn't be more explicit in his characterisation of the home to which he would always be drawn, nor more naked in his vocalisation. He's been to Palomar (north of San Diego), and he doesn't care 'who you know'; all that matters is 'who you are'. And in this especially revealing song, the dazed and confused expatriate of *Astral Weeks* at last rediscovers his place in the world, and once he finds it at the end, he seizes on it in one of the most emotional, confrontational and impassioned vocal displays of his career.

With that hard-won self-awareness now established, the narrator of Morrison's most logically sequenced album now turns his attention to his lover. 'Comfort You' is an unusually sensitive love song in which the singer encourages his lover to let out her tears like a child. He'll take her 'weight', and later, when things become too much, she can do the same for him. The sentiment of 'Comfort You' is simple but Morrison's urging of a reversion to child-like tears is again revealing. Surely

Nothing but a stranger in this world (1968–1974)

this primal, purgative release of infantile emotion is exactly what Morrison himself does in so much of his work — releasing the child within. Of all the female muses of Morrison's career, Carol Guida seems to have evoked emotions in song that he had never addressed so clearly before. In bringing him out of himself, she allowed him the opportunity for an unprecedented act of self-revelation, just as this 'American' singer's return to Ireland allowed him to understand and appreciate his own culture as never before, from an expatriate's perspective.

The same genuine, giving emotion permeates 'Come Here My Love', another deeply affecting love song which succinctly pares to its essence much of the singer's persona and many of his preoccupations. Highly introspective, it begins with the singer in melancholy mood, summoning the lover to raise his spirits. He wants to contemplate the fields and leaves, and to talk about nothing in particular. The destination of the assignation is the familiar one, namely becoming 'enraptured by the sights and sounds . . . of nature's beauty'.

In intimate, breathless tones, Van wants his lover to 'take it all in' with him. Directly expressed and filled with emotion, 'Come Here My Love' reveals a side of Morrison to which he regularly alludes, but never in such an uncomplicated and loving manner. Listening to its peaceful invocation to share in his contemplative mood, one could almost be forgiven for concluding that the singer was a nice guy. But then it's as if he becomes embarrassed by the purity of the emotion: like several tracks on this nakedly honest album, the song simply cuts out when the degree of self-confession becomes too much.

A working man in his prime

Equally moving musically, the concluding 'Country Fair' nevertheless raises an incidental smile among devotees, owing to its textbook examples of Van Morrison imagery. In verse one the singer watches the river flow, verse two finds him lying 'out in the long green grass', verse three has 'cool night air' in the summertime, and so on — all of it centred on the distinctly Irish country fair of the title. But as so often with Morrison's songs, the hackneyed lyrics (by this, his seventh album, Van was already repeating himself regularly) are merely the vehicle for the progress of the meditation. With the recorder again meandering through the song, the acoustic guitar twanging fluidly and Morrison singing well within himself, it's as if the singer is sitting on a hill looking down at the land of his birth. Haunting, timeless and ravishingly beautiful (a version of the same melody would be used many years later in 'The Mystery', from 1987's *Poetic Champions Compose*), 'Country Fair' makes a compelling conclusion not just to this final studio album before the creative hiatus, but to the entire creative journey that began six years earlier with *Astral Weeks*. Typical of much folk music in that it doesn't seek to make a 'sound' but rather expresses an inner feeling, 'Country Fair' is the song of a singer connecting with his place.

Commercially, of course, this personal reconnection with his roots was a strange phenomenon in a record industry in which spandex and hit tunes were the order of the day. The album remains an artistic triumph but a modest commercial performer, and a comparatively obscure contribution to his career as a whole. At that moment in 1974, when it seemed that Morrison had finally discovered a convincing, honest and unashamedly attractive synthesis of all the elements that make

Nothing but a stranger in this world (1968–1974)

up his musical personality, it was as if he had nothing left to offer the business in which he had worked so hard. He'd come home at last, and for quite some time thereafter the emotion of that experience would out-muscle his compulsive desire to work.

It was as if *Veedon Fleece* was an 'anti-cleaning windows' experience which had taken him outside his usual obsession with the working-day life and instead shown him who he actually was. Over the ensuing years it would drive him to books, spiritual research, occasional guest-gigging and collaborations, but the journey homeward from so far away would stop him releasing any new material for a very long time by his standards.

He would never stand so naked before his audience again. Even by the time he returned fully to this vein in *Irish Heartbeat*, fourteen years later, his gruff and disinterested demeanour acted as a disguise to his inner emotions. In those difficult years through the late 1970s he once more became a stranger in a strange land and an increasingly misanthropic figure, embittered by the 'world of lies'.

The journey towards the emotional honesty of *Veedon Fleece* had been a monumental battle that achieved many victories along the way, but had taken its toll. Once the muse returned, in subsequent years, Morrison would continue his trans-Atlantic journeys, but always with professional outcomes in mind, and rarely with such personal ambitions to discover, through music, who he actually was. He still put on his cowboy suit for a living, but no longer with the childhood thrill of imagining that it might all be true.

CRY FOR HOME
(1975–1991)

■ *A Period of Transition* ■ *Wavelength* ■ *Into the Music*
■ *Common One* ■ *Beautiful Vision* ■ *Inarticulate Speech
of the Heart* ■ *A Sense of Wonder* ■ *No Guru, No
Method, No Teacher* ■ *Poetic Champions Compose* ■ *Irish
Heartbeat* ■ *Avalon Sunset* ■ *Enlightenment* ■ *Hymns to
the Silence*

In the end, something had to give. Not even as spontaneous an artist as Van Morrison could sustain the level of creative output that saw seven complete albums of generally inspired music released in the space of six years. Ultimately, the only way for Morrison to go in 1975 was into temporary burnout.

By this stage, the themes, styles and preoccupations of the artist's future career had been established. The voice, of course, was always the focal point. No one in popular music could match him for the range of his expression or for the character embodied in his extraordinary kit-bag of vocal gestures. Increasingly in the years that followed those marvellous first seven albums, Morrison's approach to each new release has wavered between ground-breaking, unique contributions to modern music (two examples being *Common One* in 1980 and *No Guru, No Method, No Teacher* in 1986) and homage or genre-based recordings (like most of the albums from the late 1990s).

Given that Morrison worships the ground that so many of his predecessors walked on, there's no shortage of material to record, even when the songwriter himself is uninspired. But one can never be sure whether the journey with Van Morrison will lead to heaven or the vault. The miracle is that the albums released between 1977 and 1991 (thirteen studio releases and roughly 150 songs) contained so many songs of a high quality. But in them — in their philosophical and spiritual searching, in their restless parallels between sexual and mystical unions, in their handful of Top 40 hits, in their evocations of childhood, in their complaints and rants, and most of all in their tracing of the troubled journey home — they form a body of musical work which few artists who rose to fame in the 1960s can match. The journey from 1975 to 1991 started 'nowhere', in creative limbo, but it ended with Irish folk songs, Protestant hymns and Van Morrison firmly enthroned as the definitive modern Irish musician.

Along the way, the work of the jobbing musician continued at a mostly unrelenting pace, with a host of high-profile gigs. Van first appeared at the Glastonbury Festival in 1982 and in subsequent visits ('87, '89, '92, '93, '97) became something of an institution there; another high-profile live event was Roger Waters's all-star performance of *The Wall* in July 1990, by the site of the Berlin Wall, when Van with surviving members of the

A working man in his prime

Band performed 'Comfortably Numb' (released on *The Wall — Live in Berlin*). He flirted with Scientology, organised a conference on the healing power of music, and increasingly collaborated with peers, from John Lee Hooker to Cliff Richard and — the man who would become his longtime sidekick — Georgie Fame.

Yet through the changes of personnel and style, the restless search for meaning continued, and the journey toward home beckoned louder and louder.

A PERIOD OF TRANSITION
(April 1977)

- *You Gotta Make it Through the World* ▪ *It Fills You Up*
- *The Eternal Kansas City* ▪ *Joyous Sound* ▪ *Flamingos Fly*
- *Heavy Connection* ▪ *Cold Wind in August*

Van Morrison is an indiscriminate artist, it seems. One moment he's in mystical rapture, the next he's belting out some forgettable r&b filler, meaning that sometimes his prodigious gifts are at the service of inferior material and the incomparable voice is wasted in a narrow musical space that doesn't really lead very far. This frustrating process of passing a camel through the eye of a needle really began in 1977 with the release of the pointedly titled *A Period of Transition*.

Morrison had spent the three preceding years reassessing his career. And most importantly, following the release of *Veedon Fleece* in October 1974 he'd renegotiated his recording contract with Warner Bros. in order to reduce the pressure of turning out up to two albums a year. He then used part of the hiatus to move

Cry for home (1975–1991)

to England and brush up on his literary and philosophical studies, delving into Gestalt psychology and reading Yeats.

With writer's block and no particular place to go musically, the years dragged on without an album. Projects and collaborations were planned, with Jackie DeShannon, with Joe Sample from The Crusaders, with country-and-western artists among them. A spell back in California in 1975 saw him guesting on Rolling Stone Bill Wyman's second solo effort, *Stone Alone*, and taking part in his own sessions at the Record Plant (songs from which would eventually surface on *The Philosopher's Stone*); while a visit to the Band's studio in Malibu in March 1976, during the recording of Eric Clapton's *No Reason to Cry* album, seems to have lead to nothing more than Morrison helping the English guitarist celebrate his thirty-first birthday.

It was only during his fine cameo at the Band's farewell concert later that year, at San Francisco's Winterland Theater, that Morrison really seemed to commit and connect. Having performed two songs midway through the show, Van then joined Dylan, Muddy Waters, Clapton, Neil Young, Dr John et al for the rousing finale, 'I Shall Be Released'. It was the Ulsterman's first gig in two years, but to many he was the show's standout performer — drummer Levon Helm even going so far as to say he saved the night after Joni Mitchell's rather lacklustre turn. The public, however, would not get to appreciate this triumph until April 1978, when the live album and Martin Scorsese's film of the event were released.

When at last something emerged bearing Van Morrison's name, in early 1977, it was just thirty-three minutes of funk entitled *A Period of Transition*, and it arrived in the middle of the British punk rock explosion. It was probably at this moment that Morrison's reputation for hitting and missing began. Not that *A Period of Transition* is actually a bad album. On the contrary, it is — or at least it has the makings of — a fine piece of work with scarcely a bad track on it. But where previously Lewis Merenstein and Ted Templeman had peeled away the layers and added eccentric touches (dramatic cuts, unusual collaborators and musical instruments) to reveal a unique Van Morrison, here co-producer Dr John (aka Mac Rebennack) confined Morrison in a funk and gospel cage. No doubt this was never part of the plan back at the Winterland in November, when the idea for the project came up.

After two-and-a-half years of silence, fans could have been forgiven for expecting a masterpiece to emerge from Morrison's new home base in the Oxfordshire countryside. Instead they were delivered an album that was less than the sum of its parts, as if a convalescent Van had gone back to work on light duties only. Seven new tracks was what the wait was worth, at least two of which would turn out to be from earlier in the '70s, all backed by a band that never seemed to lift the singer: Dr John himself on keyboards, guitarist Marlo Henderson (later a sideman for Earth Wind & Fire and the Pointer Sisters), Rolling Stones' sideman Ollie Brown handling the drums, bassist Reggie McBride and a three-piece horn section.

In the album-opening 'You Gotta Make it Through the World', we enter, not for the first time, the territory of the Morrison complaint song. The protagonist moans that people take you for a 'clown' and 'they're bound to bring you down', and the only solution is to do what the title says. It's barely hinted at here in this half-baked lyrical effort, but the

Cry for home (1975–1991)

misanthropic genre that would dominate Morrison's music in the 1990s can trace itself back to this initial protest about the difficulty of living among unsympathetic critics.

'It Fills You Up' begins not unlike a complaint from Bob Dylan's character Mr Jones: something is going on in the world, 'but you don't know what it is'. Foreshadowing future, more mystical efforts, the song suggests that there's another realm where kings and queens dwell, but avoids references to the Arthurian world that would become prominent on subsequent albums. Instead, 'It Fills You Up' resolves into directives to 'sing with the music and groove'.

'The Eternal Kansas City' is Morrison's first extended musical homage, paying tribute not just to the American blues, jazz and big-band city but to the artists who made it famous — 'Charlie Parker, Basie and Young, Witherspoon and Jay McShann', joined later by Billie Holiday. It's a catalogue of luminaries that would become an idiosyncracy in later work, but here there's not much more to the song than this list, and the interminable repeats of the chorus. An edited version was released as a single in the UK.

Next up is 'Joyous Sound', the album's first single (and, in fact, one of the tracks recorded at the Record Plant sessions two years previously). An uncomplicated love song, the angle is simply that there's a joyous sound whenever the lovers meet, while the only distinctive feature is the promise that 'grace will follow us'. When Van meets a girl, it often prompts him to piety.

'Flamingos Fly' is another love song, in which the destination is 'way over yonder in the clear blue sky'. (It's also another song from the past, dating back to the Jackie DeShannon sessions in 1973 and Morrison's in Hilversum the following year.) Wherever that place is exactly, it's a veritable aviary, featuring not only the flamingos of the title but also the lark and the nightingale. Before this idea is developed, however, the singer finds himself talking instead about taking a road back home, and this time the wildlife consists of 'deer and the provincial angels'. While the imagery is confused, the emotion isn't, with the lover explicitly filling the singer with happiness.

Although its lyrics are no more profound, 'Heavy Connection' is a rather more typical Morrison song, beginning in 'the land of a thousand dances' — the dancing metaphor survived the creative dry patch — and with the lovers separated in different countries. There are references to Amsterdam and Hamburg's Reeperbahn, but again the ideas remain underdeveloped and the song resolves in repeats of the chorus, 'la-la-la's and 'baby-baby-baby's.

And finally there's 'Cold Wind in August', which finds the lover absent altogether, while the protagonist shivers in the rain waiting for his erotic Godot under a 'California pine'. The only other thing to say about 'Cold Wind in August' is that, coupled with 'Moondance' on a single, it gave the 1970 classic a belated run on the US chart.

So, *A Period of Transition* contains some sketchy pointers to future directions and no real stinkers (although the sub–'Snow in San Anselmo' choir on 'The Eternal Kansas City' does its best to ruin an already-problematic piece). In concert, Morrison would continue to revisit numbers like 'It Fills You Up' for decades afterwards, which says something for his commitment to these songs, but there are no standout tracks and nothing except the inimitable voice to take the listener's breath away. Still, at least the artist and record company managed to get something out to end the creative hiatus, it's just that there's not enough of it and nor is it of sufficient quality to satisfy those who know Morrison as the genius behind *Astral Weeks* and *Saint Dominic's Preview*.

It would actually be 1980 before Van Morrison truly risked creative failure again with a groundbreaking album. In the meantime, *A Period of Transition* opened the way for two further albums of standard-format, mainly American-style repertoire as the artist — going through profound personal change via divorce, self-education and restless crossings of the Atlantic — sought to rebuild his identity within the confines of a music industry reeling from the onslaught of punk.

WAVELENGTH

(September 1978)

■ *Kingdom Hall* ■ *Checkin' it Out* ■ *Natalia* ■ *Venice USA* ■ *Lifetimes* ■ *Wavelength* ■ *Santa Fe / Beautiful Obsession* ■ *Hungry For Your Love* ■ *Take it Where You Find it*

Although the singer had changed the terms of his contract with Warners to allow him more time between albums, Van Morrison's follow-up to *A Period of Transition* was ready in just over a year. In the interim, his stock had been raised significantly by the release of *The Last Waltz*, the film document of the Band's all-star send-off, and he'd also returned to the concert stage, in mid 1978, beginning what would be his first major tour for over four years.

His live band was made up of the same musicians that had just taken part in the sessions for his new album, *Wavelength*.

A working man in his prime

But, unlike the funky studio cats assembled by Dr John, some of Morrison's players this time actually had a history with the singer. The links with guitarist Herbie Armstrong and keyboard player Pete Bardens, for instance, went way back to Belfast and the '60s, Bardens being a member of Them at one point; while Garth Hudson's guest spots on keyboards recalled the happy times with the Band up at Woodstock. More recently, drummer Peter van Hooke was there at the sessions in Hilversum, when Van stopped by with some of the musicians who backed him at Montreux in June 1974.

The result of this union was a slick, West Coast album of pop songs, and the polish even seems to have rubbed off on the singer, judging by his dapper appearance on the cover. But *Wavelength* displays signs of sewing together the threads of Morrison's mystical research during the years of hiatus. It's an album that tentatively re-examines his own identity, placing the self within the ambit of a larger force.

This is true right from the outset, on the opening 'Kingdom Hall'. In music that sounds distinctly American, Morrison nevertheless recounts his childhood encounters with the Jehovah's Witness sect at the Kingdom Hall in Belfast. And what a swinging encounter it is, bringing an upbeat mood that never really leaves during this album, even in the meditative, highly revealing conclusion to side one, 'Lifetimes'.

This latter song begins familiarly enough. The lover is first seen, like so many before and after her, standing down by the river, and the narrator has come (*Veedon Fleece*-style) to calm her fears. But as the song proceeds — and the water images of rivers flowing and boatmen singing across the water proliferate — Morrison begins to play with time. The lover

Cry for home (1975–1991)

has been known not just in this lifetime but in previous ones also, and the answer to current troubles can be found in feeling the silence and listening to 'the music inside'. It's a critical trope in Morrison's work, this notion that silence is something felt while hearing is an internal sense.

Other tracks on this unpretentious album also bop their way along with incidental reference to crucial themes. 'Natalia' begins down on the 'lonely avenue', and in amidst the 'na na na's of the catchy chorus we gather that the singer wants to pick up Natalia so that they can go walking together. Evidently, as dozens of songs testify, to be Morrison's lover, a woman must own a stout pair of shoes.

'Checkin' it Out' (track two, preceding 'Natalia') confronts the obstacles of life with 'guides and spirits . . . who befriend us'. To solve problems with another, the singer wants to 'get into it' across the table 'like a meditation'. The sound is as Californian as the New Age mentality on display — Van in feel-good, vegetarian mode.

'Venice USA', the other song on side one, has the chorus 'Dum derra dum dum diddy diddy dah dah' but more significantly involves a walk down by the harbour, where Morrison sees 'the ships comes sailing in' (as he would do again many years later in the company of John Lee Hooker). Garth Hudson's accordion adds to the seafront imagery.

Morrison's head voice returns for one of the final times in his career on the title track. Starting slowly, 'Wavelength' then settles into its Fleetwood Mac-style groove accompanied by a whirling synthesizer obbligato and even a genuine electric guitar solo! More importantly, this title song is all about returning to America after the singer's adopted nation had called out to him on the radio. The wavelength of the title refers to the radio signal — the sound of America that had inspired Morrison throughout his life, beckoning him over the Atlantic and resulting here in one of the most 'American' studio sounds he would ever create. Strangely enough, the American vision of 'Wavelength' was actually created in Richard Branson's studio in Oxfordshire.

'Santa Fe' opens in familiar lyrical territory, with 'train wheels runnin' down an open track', inspiring thoughts of going back in time, and with memories of the past emerging from everyday situations. Co-written with Jackie DeShannon (and dating back to their 1973 sessions together), the memories become 'more than a song to sing', although the personal significance of the lyric is evidently more urgent to the writers than to the listener. A rather pedestrian track, 'Santa Fe' is most notable for its seamless segue into 'Beautiful Obsession', which is scarcely more intelligible at the literal level, and shares the 'more than a song to sing' lyric. More interesting is the use of the phrase 'Let the cowboy ride' as the concluding mantra, a variation on the 'hi ho, Silver's and 'Geronimo's found on *Veedon Fleece*.

'Hungry For Your Love' is a self-explanatory song of separated lovers, made more intriguing by the fantasy line 'I love you in buckskin'. It's *Annie Get Your Gun* with Morrison apparently still keen to get girls to join in on his childhood cowboy games.

This childlike vision is developed in the final, epic track, 'Take it Where You Find it'. Here, the songwriter reflects the reading that he'd been doing over preceding years. A song about philosophical wonder, it muses on the great mysteries

Cry for home (1975–1991)

('stars at the edge of the sea', 'thoughts about liberty'). The ambition is to find a purpose to carry on, and Morrison does this by seeing the world 'through the eyes of a child'. The attitude to America is now ambivalent: it's a place, explicitly, of 'lost dreams and found dreams', where you have to discover what is real and what can genuinely sustain the individual caught in a complex free society.

And then, after three verses spent pondering these weighty and uncharacteristically sophisticated issues, a miraculous change comes over the music as Morrison decides that he's going to 'walk down the street' in pursuit of his own 'shining light'. It's a transcendental moment in an otherwise commercially hidebound album, and one of the most uplifting transitions in all of Morrison's recorded music. 'Take it Where You Find it' is a triumphant conclusion to a significant spiritual journey, and a positive statement of identity in a pop world where the negativity of punk and the brainlessness of disco almost demanded that great artists should take a different tack and say something important.

On this glorious concluding track to *Wavelength*, Morrison did just that, and it's curious that 'Take it Where You Find it' has never been highly regarded by his biographers. Perhaps it's because its inspiring lyrics and its self-aware attitude are diametrically opposed to the 'standard' vision of Morrison — the miserable, name-dropping, curmudgeonly old dilettante who only dabbles in self-knowledge as a means to furnish a lyric. In time it may come to be seen as one of his greatest songs.

The pleasant, disciplined sound on *Wavelength* was no doubt designed to ensure wide airplay for its three singles (the title track, 'Natalia' and 'Kingdom Hall'), and sure enough his ninth album returned Morrison to the Top 30 on the American album chart for the first time since *Hard Nose the Highway* five years before. But generally, from this period on, it would be in Britain that Van Morrison most caught the imagination of the record-buying public. His tour would reach there early in 1979, the time on the road allowing Morrison to build on the chemistry and dynamics of his new band. The result of this would be one of the highlights of his next, far more confident collection of songs.

INTO THE MUSIC
(August 1979)

▪ Bright Side of the Road ▪ Full Force Gale ▪ Stepping Out Queen ▪ Troubadours ▪ Rolling Hills ▪ You Make Me Feel So Free ▪ Angelou ▪ And the Healing Has Begun ▪ It's All in the Game / You Know What They're Writing About

It took Van Morrison many years of dedicated reading and research to come up with the ideas contained in the lyrics of his tenth album, his first for Mercury (although Warner Bros. would continue to be his distributor in America until 1984). The music side, however, would take him just twelve months, building on the band he'd assembled for *Wavelength*.

Gathering at the Record Plant in Sausalito, Marin County, were a mix of old faces and new. Herbie Armstrong and Peter van Hooke, on guitar and drums respectively, and singer Katie Kissoon stayed on after the tour, while new in were Tony Marcus (on mandolin, violin and viola), Pee Wee

Cry for home (1975–1991)

Ellis (James Brown's longtime sideman, on sax) and Mark Isham (on trumpet). Returning to the fold were bassist David Hayes and pianist Mark Jordan, both of whom had regularly backed Morrison earlier in the '70s and had taken part in the apparently fruitless Record Plant sessions in 1975.

At around this time, down at the legendary Muscle Shoals Sound Studios in Alabama, Bob Dylan was recording *Slow Train Coming*, an album that would herald the dawn of a new phase in his professional career and personal life. In songs of great piety and little musical interest, the Jewish-born Bob announced with Old Testament certainty that he was now a born-again Christian.

Come August, in the very same week that *Slow Train Coming* fell on the deaf or cynical ears of most of the world's music critics, Van Morrison released *Into the Music*, in which not dissimilar Christian sentiments popped up at crucial moments. The presence of pious homilies ('I will always return to the Lord', 'I will find my sanctuary in the Lord', 'I was lifted up again by the Lord', 'I will live my life in Him', 'I will read my Bible still among the rolling hills') in Morrison's new work passed relatively unnoticed, however. In part this was because, unlike with Dylan, the blatantly Christian references were not the substance of the album as a whole but confined to just two songs, 'Full Force Gale' and 'Rolling Hills'.

Morrison's music — or at least his lyrics — had always embraced a devotional element, not necessarily paying homage to Christianity per se but to musical idols, nature and the power of meditation, and so the shift into explicit Christian references was hardly dramatic. The fact that the two 'Christian' songs were offset by alternative references to 'dharma' (in 'Stepping

Out Queen') only reinforced the breadth of Morrison's 'Christianity'; he was a bower-bird collecting whatever he could from individual religions and theories, rather than a fanatical evangelist proselytising the benefits of any one way of thought. He was, in short, a rather more sophisticated and perhaps better-read religious rock star than those trapped in the narrow confines of a single cult or doctrine.

More importantly, where Dylan's Christianity represented the nadir of an already problematic career, *Into the Music* was a stunning return to form. Conceived as a suite of strong songs, it moves from the buoyant and bubbly opening tracks 'Bright Side of the Road' (the album's single, complete with Louis Armstrong impersonation) and 'Full Force Gale' (sounding like an adaptation of Elvis Presley's 'Burning Love', with a tidy slide-guitar solo from Ry Cooder), through other good-time tunes such as 'You Make Me Feel So Free', to the seamless, meditative transitions that constitute the hypnotic and beautiful final third of the album. With the vocals keening, shouted, spoken, growled and husked, there is perhaps no better album with which to introduce a novice into the diverse, thrilling, exasperating and uniquely rewarding music of Van Morrison.

For once, the album's title actually reflects the content. Each track pushes ever deeper, from funk to folk and then on to the epic interior monologues of 'And the Healing Has Begun' and 'It's All in the Game'. The latter song is a cover but, with Morrison's interpolations of 'You Know What They're Writing About' and speaking-in-tongues vocal elaborations, it's almost another original.

We enter more and more not just into the music, but into the mind of its creator. And the deeper we go, and the more

Cry for home (1975–1991)

internalised *Into the Music* becomes, the more 'space' appears to emerge in the music. This journey into self — which the album essentially is — is a revelation of timelessness and infinity, a world of possibilities and exquisite beauty where everything opens up just as it becomes most intimate.

The overt Christianity had been brewing since childhood, of course, but new ideas were beginning to emerge too, and Morrison had already demonstrated — as the run-through of styles and genres on *Into the Music* celebrates so virtuosically — that he only had one real religion, and that was music itself. This was the album where the songwriter first introduced the idea of music as a healing force, perhaps the single most important trope that he would pursue both in song and also offstage during his subsequent career, reaching a climax in his 1997 album, *The Healing Game*. 'And the Healing Has Begun' occupies a crucial position in his work, not just because it inaugurates the music-therapy message (gleaned from writers and theorists such as Elizabeth Clare Prophet and Cyril Scott), but also because it is one of the most successful examples of Morrison 'riding a groove' from the here and now into something approaching spiritual ecstasy. It demonstrates in music the kind of sublime transformation into a state of spiritual grace that Dylan could only talk about second-hand, in his explicitly 'religious' lyrics.

This quintessential Van Morrison song begins with a nod to Irving Berlin and a 'walk down the avenue', while the songs he hears being sung emerge not from a distant radio but 'from way back when'. Although it's barely noticeable in its embryonic form here, all that reading and discussion about mysticism, spirituality and philosophy that Morrison had been undertaking during his professional sabbatical was beginning to turn up in lyrics such as this, where the source of power was no longer just childhood but a much more distant and evocative antiquity. From this time onwards, the word 'ancient' would appear at significant moments in his lyrics, filling the contemporary searcher with hope and light — the kind of hope and light that form the central imagery of *Into the Music* itself.

In this particular incarnation, 'the songs from way back when' are 'the music of the soul' that is prompted by hearing 'backstreet rock 'n' roll' — not even the most in-your-face art form ever created can be entirely externalised in this hymn to self. It's from the backstreets, not to mention the back-catalogues. We're in the world of 'Caravan' once more, but now with a more informed historical sense as we head outside 'underneath the stars' and have another one of those campfire singalongs, accompanied on this occasion by 'violin and the two guitars'. Staying 'out all night' doing this leaves only two inevitable Morrison tasks to be achieved: dancing and a little backstreet jellyroll.

These lyrics straight from the Morrison kit-bag are only a means to an end, however. The point of 'And the Healing Has Begun' is the healing generated through the music and the performance. And as the folksy accompaniment proceeds, cutting back only for the spoken middle section (where Van seduces his woman after a gig, with Muddy Waters playing on the stereo), the ebb and flow of the song becomes mesmeric, creating its own sense of time. Somehow, what appears on paper as a simple and clear structure is irrelevant.

Although the album was written in Oxfordshire and

recorded in California, its subtext is always Ireland. With the jig-like 'Rolling Hills', ever-present fiddles and violas (given a Curved Air-style workout on 'Stepping Out Queen') and the celebration of the ancient 'Troubadours', through to the participation of tin-whistler, fellow spiritual searcher and all-round folk hero Robin Williamson, this is the first album that links the Irish folk leanings of *Veedon Fleece* with the Celtic reality of *Irish Heartbeat*.

But there would be much more in between these explicit moments of Celtic musical excavation, and the creative riches contained in *Into the Music* extend beyond Christianity, time travel and folk music. In this album, specifically in 'Stepping Out Queen', the phrase 'in the garden' makes a notable debut, being a place where the lovers can look at the flowers and just 'talk for hours and hours'. This garden imagery, together with the repeated references to Paris in May in 'Angelou' — not to mention the downright joyful music of the album's first half — make *Into the Music* a 'springtime' album through and through. It bursts with love of life and the excitement of intellectual discovery, and, as such, truly was the comeback album that *A Period of Transition* could never be and *Wavelength* almost was.

COMMON ONE
(August 1980)

- *Haunts of Ancient Peace* ▪ *Summertime in England*
- *Satisfied* ▪ *Wild Honey* ▪ *Spirit* ▪ *When Heart Is Open*

Once Van Morrison had entered the contemplative world at the end of *Into the Music*, it was as if he had no desire to

A working man in his prime

leave. Even so, nothing could have prepared fans for *Common One* — still the most hotly debated and perhaps most critically reviled of all his albums.

Its recording took place at Super Bear in the French Alps during an intense nine-day recording session in February, his band little changed from the last album, save for the fact that John Allair took over on keyboards and violinist Tony Marcus had departed. An unusual location for Morrison to choose to record in, it was as if the singer was looking down from a mountain-top like some lonely ascetic surveying the world below through the rising mist.

Whereas his previous releases are characterised by attention-grabbing, often quite upbeat openings, the first bars of 'Haunts of Ancient Peace' announce that *Common One* is going to be a very different, decidedly uncommercial album. Over a haunting, hushed accompaniment of Fender Rhodes and bass, Mark Isham's muted trumpet weaves an arabesque with no particular end in mind, the music emerging as if out of distant memory. The destination of *Into the Music* has become the departure point for *Common One*. As though to emphasise the point that we are no longer dancing a jig among the 'Rolling Hills', the first track even has Pee Wee Ellis's saxophone pose the question 'How Are Things in Glocca Morra?', as it quotes the hit song from the Irish-kitsch musical *Finian's Rainbow*.

Never had the objectives of peace and silence been attempted so unequivocally in Morrison's work, resulting in incomprehension and derision from a sceptical musical establishment. With the first two numbers sprawling over a total of twenty-three minutes, with 'Haunts of Ancient Peace'

Cry for home (1975–1991)

intentionally having no real rhythmic drive whatsoever, and with the multi-part 'Summertime in England' shifting between four and three beats in the bar, this was largely hook-free music designed for meditation and contemplation. There were no singles to be found on the album. Morrison was essentially a hit-maker whose opening tracks ('And It Stoned Me', 'Domino', 'Wild Night', 'Jackie Wilson Said' and 'Bright Side of the Road') were radio-friendly three-minute songs that might be repeated ad infinitum. But this commercial side to Morrison was only one aspect of a complex musical personality. On *Common One*, he demonstrated the other side, which was not only original — indeed unique — but would furnish the aesthetics of virtually all his albums released during the 1980s.

To the devotee looking to experience the essential creative genius of Van Morrison, *Common One* is an album to speak about in hushed tones. While not as consistently inspired as the later masterpiece *No Guru, No Method, No Teacher* (a work that shares and develops many of the themes and ideas from *Common One*), there is no question that it represents a turning point in the singer's career. This was the album in which Van at last sought explicitly to marry the past with the present, where the ghosts of Mahalia Jackson and William Blake step hand-in-hand out of some distant antiquity, where Jesus walks on ancient English soil, and where the haunting presence of Stonehenge seems to hover in the background of every note played.

Undoubtedly the constant name-dropping in 'Summertime in England' has contributed to the album's hostile critical reception ('hopelessly self-indulgent', according to Patrick Humphries in his 1997 analysis of Morrison's work; 'insulting to anyone to whom the great poets matter' in John Collis's strident opinion). Nevertheless, it's odd to realise that Morrison is rarely criticised for singing no lyrics at all, and yet when he makes reference to more literary subject matter, he's whacked on the head for being an intellectual clod! True, 'Did you ever hear about Wordsworth and Coleridge, baby? / They were smokin' up in Kendal' is an appalling couple of lines, but in the context of the fifteen-minute epic in which they appear, they form a failed part of an heroic act of musical exploration. That bit doesn't come off, but much more of 'Summertime in England' does. Not the best but perhaps the quintessential Morrison song, it has become a staple in the singer's live sets, jeopardised not so much by the Lake Poets couplet as by the constant (and constantly irritating) call-and-response routines that he and his back-up vocalists engage in during it.

So what is this extraordinary world that Morrison creates in his most challenging and brave album? Essentially it's a search for 'harmony and rhyme' — not the makings of a song but the coherence and balance that can be achieved within a contemplative life. As stated in the opening lyrics, the search is for love and light, a place where mere words are no longer required. This impressionistic depiction of the English countryside has diverse counterparts in the modal pastoralism of Vaughan Williams, in Mike Oldfield's *Hergest Ridge* (the latter created in the same Oxfordshire studio that Morrison had worked in during preparations for the album) and in Thomas Hardy's depiction in the opening chapter of *The Return of the Native* of the windswept heath a hundred miles to the south-west. Indeed, the cover of *Common One*, with its peasant-like human figure struggling up an exposed rural hill looks like a cross between a Led Zeppelin backdrop and a filmed image from Hardy's Wessex. Perhaps it's Van himself on Glastonbury Tor, or Hardy's reddleman crossing the moors. Maybe it's just an ancient everyman — the 'common one' of the title.

Beyond the cover art and into the music, it's a Blakean landscape tinged with echoes of Arthurian legend. Here the Holy Grail that is being sought amid the country towns and ringing Sunday church bells is actually Blake's New Jerusalem. The importance of this setting shouldn't be underestimated, coming as it does from an artist often wrongly associated with rock 'n' roll. At the end of 'Haunts of Ancient Peace' he whispers, 'Be still.' This is no rock star. This is a man on a spiritual search, through the past, for peace and eternal truths, the rewards for a life lived beyond words in stillness and contemplation.

Just as the ultimate ambition of Morrison's musical performances is silence, so his thematic preoccupation is a world devoid of fashion. It's an ancient world in which the trends of the moment are fleeting images set against a monumental backdrop of mystical grandeur and historical power that — like the image on the album cover — see the individual dwarfed against, and yet inspired by, the forces of history and national identity.

There is nothing more anti-rock 'n' roll than these images of timelessness and historical currency of ancient ideals. Heavy metal music, of course, with its penchant for screen-printed images of Norse gods, has often broached this territory, but in nothing like the considered, well-read and frankly lucid manner in which Morrison does it here. The riffs of soul music seek to establish links with a distant world of legends and heroes, and whether it succeeds or fails (and history may prove that it does more of the former than the latter), the importance of the attempt to bring together two worlds in harmony deserves plaudits. With the possible exception of *No Guru*, no album so emphatically demonstrates that away from the demands of the commercial popular music industry, Morrison is at heart a mystic.

The intellectual weight of the album falls on those first two songs (an entire album side), but the preoccupations and spiritual quest are present throughout the remainder as well. The funky, upbeat, sax-squealing character of 'Satisfied' sounds like he's satisfied, but the song's lyrics speak of spiritual doubt. It begins with a walk up a mountain-side to 'survey this wondrous scene' — a microcosmic depiction of the album as a whole — and announces that the singer is satisfied with his world because *he* 'made it the way it is'. (Interestingly, there is no God or guru here.) But it's a world of 'spiritual hunger and spiritual thirst' that has to be changed 'on the inside first'. The important lines are 'Sometimes I think I know where it's at [/how it is] / Other times I'm completely in the dark'. If this is the answer to the Rolling Stones' '(I Can't Get No) Satisfaction', then it's a highly uncomfortable one. Enlightenment is just an eye-flicker from extinction.

The image of the mountain-top also permeates 'Wild Honey'. The singer will wait there for his love, in that lofty place where 'the light comes shining through'. His heart is beating fast in anticipation of the lover's arrival; spiritual and sexual ecstasy just around the corner, as the lonely Romantic exile looks down on a world of confusion. An inspiring vantage

Cry for home (1975–1991)

point at the time, it could never be sustained in its entirety. And even though the lofty mountain-top was always the preferred vantage point, in years to come the writer of these ecstatic lyrics would return with increasing frequency to whinges about the sharks and big-time operators of the music industry.

'Spirit' was a hangover from the *Into the Music* sessions and is another uplifting number, born out of feelings of despair but then leaping into life in the chorus, with the homily to 'never let spirit die'. You get out, you follow the road, you get back home. In a superficially trivial lyric, Morrison writes autobiography with explicit force and considerable emotional depth. Nothing much in itself — indeed the formulaic musical nature of the track means that it might easily be passed over on a cursory listen — it is nevertheless a summary of his career and an essential, positive component of the composer's self-mythology.

And then we have the fifteen-minute track that always causes the most furore in debates about the merits of *Common One*. 'When Heart Is Open' begins like something from the Doors' 'The End', with Indian raga sounds and keening, but no real rhythm track. It might be better suited to a meditation instruction tape. John Collis describes it as 'impossible to listen to' and 'the worst song he ever released', but it's much less appalling than that. In fact, with its distant, Irish-sounding wind instruments (not tin whistles and uillean pipes yet, but they soon would be) and extended keening, this is the song that Van Morrison was always destined to record. Eight years before his collaboration with the Chieftains, 'When Heart Is Open' was where the Irish roots of his art were laid bare, with lyrics of no particular distinction or consequence, ending in whispers — a land without words.

A working man in his prime

To describe it as a weak track is to pigeonhole Morrison and to turn one's back on the Irish tradition that sustains him even when he is at his most 'American'. Ravishing and spellbinding, 'When Heart Is Open' finds the singer at his most personal and private. Like so much else on *Common One*, if it fails, it does so nobly, in pursuit of an authentic voice.

BEAUTIFUL VISION
(February 1982)

■ *Celtic Ray* ■ *Northern Muse (Solid Ground)* ■ *Dweller on the Threshold* ■ *Beautiful Vision* ■ *She Gives Me Religion* ■ *Cleaning Windows* ■ *Vanlose Stairway* ■ *Aryan Mist* ■ *Across the Bridge Where Angels Dwell* ■ *Scandinavia* [instrumental]

The pull of home became stronger with each album Van Morrison released. Ever since *Veedon Fleece* captured the holiday snapshot of Ireland, moments in all the subsequent albums made incidental or tangential reference to the land of his birth, with keening in the vocals and the occasional whistle or uillean pipes in the band. By *Into the Music* in 1979, entire songs (like 'Rolling Hills') began to make reference to the Irish folk tradition. But the confessional nature of the ever-so-British *Common One* had opened the door to a whole new world — or rather old world — and its successor was to be a collection fixated on the theme of homecoming.

Recorded in 1981 at a time when Morrison was relocating permanently back to the British Isles, *Beautiful Vision* celebrates what the singer would soon afterwards call 'the cry for home'.

Cry for home (1975–1991)

Surprisingly then, it's another Sausalito album, made with the same musicians as *Common One*, the only significant change being Chris Michie's arrival as lead guitarist. Even though there are plenty of synthesizers and funk grooves among its generally solid selection of tracks, the album 'sounds' more Irish than anything — even *Veedon Fleece* — that the artist had recorded up until this point.

The meaning of the opening track, 'Celtic Ray', couldn't be more clear. Its chorus depicts Ireland, Scotland, England and Wales ringing out with mothers' voices crying, 'Children, children, children'. With these calls for homecoming singing the expatriate sons and daughters back to shore, the song is like a flip-side or completion of the traditional narrative of 'Danny Boy' — the mother no longer farewelling the departing child but calling back the lost generations of the diaspora. And Van himself is swept up in the tide, explicitly announcing, 'I want to go home'. Given the hints of an impending return home and allusions to Ireland in several previous albums, the significance of this repeated line (addressed to one 'Jimmy') shouldn't be underestimated. It's intensified by the equally direct admission that the singer has 'been away too long'.

And go home he does on this striking album, not just to Ireland but also to his spiritual home, in a series of the most overtly 'religious' lyrics he would ever write. In a mystical dog's breakfast of spiritual fervour, he invokes Alice Bailey, Krishna and the *Bhagavad-Gita* in equal measure and indulges in terminology like 'glamour', 'ray' and 'burning ground', terms which, to be understood fully, require a specialist knowledge of the esoteric writings from which they emanate.

A working man in his prime

The thinking behind a 'ray' is something like a cross between the Renaissance theory of the humours and modern-day astrology. Each of the planets emanates its own particular ray, which bestows a certain kind of enlightenment and behavioural pattern on its subjects, who can include not just individuals but entire nations. Traditionally, the Celtic, or Green, Ray is associated with the planet Venus, bestowing creativity, artistry and a rare appreciation of beauty on the Celts. In Morrison's song 'Celtic Ray', the vocals are relaxed, but there is also an apocalyptic urgency about the message. As we watch market-men — (the presumably Welsh) Llewellyn, (the presumably Irish) McManus and a 'coal-brick man' — going about their daily rounds, we're warned about the imminent arrival of the Celtic Ray and asked if we're ready for it. By the end of the song, Van himself, who had started as the one being called back, now becomes the voice of the calling: 'Come home children / Come home on the Celtic Ray'.

The call possesses a poignancy and a sense of personal grounding that are at the opposite extreme to Morrison's American soul impersonations. While not belittling his gifts as a soul singer — for there is surely no greater white interpreter of this repertoire on the planet — songs as deeply personal and confessional as 'Celtic Ray' place this 'Irish' strand of Morrison's creative personality in a league of its own. And it was this call to Irishmen everywhere (soon to be repeated in *Inarticulate Speech of the Heart*) that undoubtedly inspired a generation of Irish popular musicians, including U2, Sinead O'Connor and the Pogues. Indeed, there's some justification in suggesting that, post-*Beautiful Vision*, identifiably Irish 'citizens of the world' were at the forefront of popular music endeavour during the 1980s.

'Northern Muse (Solid Ground)' continues the Irish fixation, and the subtitle is significant. In some ways a standard love song, 'Northern Muse' is notable for its almost worshipful attitude to the Irish earth. It's almost as if Van is the Pope, kissing the ground on his arrival at the hallowed land. The lover in question hails from County Down — the county that would also provide the opening love interest in the *Irish Heartbeat* album several years later. But not forgetting his peer Bob Dylan — whose own early music often made use of Irish folk themes — Morrison builds in a refrain of 'If you see her, say hello', straight out of *Blood on the Tracks*.

The most complex track on the album in terms of its references to spiritual writings is 'Dweller on the Threshold'. The song reworks ideas from Alice Bailey's book *Glamour: A World Problem*, published in 1950 and one of approximately nineteen books that were supposedly dictated to her telepathically by a Tibetan monk, Djwal Khul. The 'glamour' in question would be described by Rastafarians as Babylon: the illusory desires, lusts and assorted trappings of the material world that keep humanity in thrall and prevent true spiritual searchers from achieving their goals on the astral plane. In Bailey's metaphor, 'glamour' is like a fog or a mist, clouding the vision, distorting the truth, and — in an argument not unlike Plato's in his theory of art — making the image obscure the ideal reality that it's meant to depict.

The purpose of the 'anti-glamour' devotee is to remove these intermediary and distracting images of the truth to get to the thing itself, which is exactly what Morrison seeks to do in so much of his singing by eschewing the specific and literal words and noise in an effort to reach the truer world of wordlessness and silence. And when that spiritual state is achieved, the teachings tell of a cataclysmic fire that burns away all the old illusions and the old foundations of belief that have previously held the searcher in thrall. This ritual act of purification goes by the term 'burning ground', a phrase that Morrison uses first in 'Dweller on the Threshold' and which then becomes the title of an entire song fifteen years later on *The Healing Game*.

The 'Dweller on the Threshold' of the title is that figure poised on the brink of enlightenment, waiting at the door for the ascent into spiritual empowerment. With typical Morrison urgency, though, this searcher is becoming impatient and doesn't want to wait anymore — perhaps the reason why this most mystical of rock stars has never subscribed fully to any one particular religion or cult. But he makes his debt to Alice Bailey clear, both in the lines 'Let me pierce the realm of glamour / So I know just who I am' and when a 'mighty crystal fire' consumes his 'darkness'. The moment of epiphany comes when he turns to face 'the music of the spheres' (a medieval and Renaissance trope much favoured by Shakespeare), when he is lifted up and darkness and midnight disappear. But the crucial lines come later, when the protagonist crosses 'the burning ground' and then goes down to the water to watch 'the great illusion drown'. Glamour is destroyed and with the path now clear to that phenomenal moment of enlightenment, the searcher nevertheless is still (in occult terms) dwelling on the threshold, and growing more impatient by the moment.

Cry for home (1975–1991)

Sophisticated listeners might hear in this most articulate of Van Morrison songs something more than the simple exploration of some dubious occult-based faith. They may hear the spiritual dissatisfaction of a man who desperately wants personal answers to the great mysteries but to whom the organised or cult-based faiths can only lead to the threshold, not to the enlightenment itself. On the evidence of songs such as 'Dweller on the Threshold', Morrison is no atheist, but neither is he a believer. He is an agnostic, and a mere step away from 'Dweller on the Threshold' is the definitive Morrison album title *No Guru, No Method, No Teacher*.

On one level the song 'Beautiful Vision' is a simple profession of love, but lines like 'You are shining bright / You are my guiding light' also imply a more mystical level. Indeed, in few other songs does Van Morrison create such an equation between physical heterosexual love and the path to spiritual enlightenment. Here, in the title track to this important album, the two are indistinguishable, and the same parallel is drawn more clearly in the song that follows.

The hit-sounding and eminently engaging 'She Gives Me Religion' is about sex and spirituality, all rolled into one, with the title saying it all. It is, of course, the popular musician's ultimate way to introduce philosophy into an art form based on carnal desire — make the quest for enlightenment parallel the search for a little backstreet jellyroll. Back in 1966, who would have thought that the stocky, snarling, spitting, screaming little front man of Them would achieve it so much better than anyone else?

The presence of the blatantly autobiographical 'Cleaning Windows' on *Beautiful Vision* has often raised eyebrows. Led by Mark Knopfler's guitar and marking a return by drummer Gary Malabar, its funky groove appears to be somewhat incongruous with the Celtic-inspired meditations that make up the other tracks (even if it made 'Cleaning Windows' the logical choice for a single). But this most revealing of Van Morrison songs, complete with its catalogue of childhood influences, is precisely the sort of material dealt with (albeit at the spiritual level) elsewhere on the album. *Beautiful Vision* is all about the spiritual search undertaken by Morrison, and it is essential that the musings about, and adolescent readings of, 'Christmas Humphreys' book on Zen' and 'Kerouac's *Dharma Bums* and *On the Road*' get a mention. After all, *Beautiful Vision* marks a journey towards — not the arrival at — a spiritual destination. The journey started with Leadbelly and Blind Lemon Jefferson, and continued through Alice Bailey, but the only end point that is reached is that of nationalism and a return to Ireland.

The sequence of songs is not necessarily the most logical, and doesn't reflect the journey. 'Cleaning Windows' might have come first on the album, for instance, followed by the Bailey songs, the love songs (and instrumental 'Scandinavia') to his current girlfriend Ulla Munch, and then the equations between physical love and spiritual enlightenment. The ideal conclusion would've been the theme of returning to Ireland, whose cry for its children carries more emotional power than any other philosophy or spiritual concept on this deep, heartfelt and articulate collection.

'Vanlose Stairway' was destined to become a staple in live sets; indeed, this track and five others from the album would make up the majority of Morrison's 1984 concert album, *Live at the Grand Opera House, Belfast.* The song fits the profile of *Beautiful Vision* perfectly, and in particular aligns with 'She Gives Me Religion' and the title track. In his lover's Danish hometown, Van stares up a set of apartment-block steps and in his imagination they become a stairway to heaven. Physically, he wants to smell her pillow and possess her copies of the Bible and the *Bhagavad-Gita*. Spiritually, he wants to take the stairway 'right up to the moon' and to 'come right back' to his lover. Religion and sex again: the same act, and the same kind of popular music to accompany them both. If there is any one single feature that sets Van Morrison apart from other popular musicians and songwriters (aside, of course, from the quality of his voice), it is surely this simultaneous extension of the traditional love song into the language of spiritual quest.

But after the last of three such songs on the album, we're back in the world of Alice Bailey for the rousing 'Aryan Mist'. The function of the word 'Aryan' in Bailey's cosmology is different from the reviled one of the Nazis. Bailey's Aryans are in fact 'the fifth race', which includes Hindus as well as Europeans and Americans, and they are no more enlightened or superior than anyone else — rather, they too suffer illusions (i.e. 'glamour') at both the physical and astral planes. They are, in short, in the 'mist', unable to find enlightenment because of the fog of illusion that surrounds them.

In Van Morrison's song, the afflicted Aryan soul hangs 'by the river' and has done so 'forever'. He asks this troubled soul if they're lifted up in this 'world full of glamour', or whether it's merely 'railway carriage charm'. This latter reference is to the drug speed, which the band Them took to keep them going during eighteen long months of touring.

The pills were referred to by the band as 'railway carriages', but of course they offered no real salvation — they were simply alternative forms of 'glamour'.

In this same song, the most obvious precursor to *No Guru, No Method, No Teacher* comes with Morrison's reference to 'gurus from the east' and 'gurus from the west' as being among the 'glamour'. Clearly this is no album championing the teachings of Alice Bailey, Djwal Khul or anyone else. The questioning of spiritual gurus is already here in Morrison's most unequivocally 'religious' album, quite plain, embodying a healthy scepticism that is likely to turn on any sophist or fake guide to nirvana. Van Morrison's interest in alternative religions proves itself to be rather more mature — and vastly more sceptical — than that of other 'spiritual celebrities'. Like the dweller on the threshold, the spiritual searcher of 'Aryan Mist' is waiting there down by the river forever, where Van wishes to be reminded of Krishna and then kissed as the interminable wait continues.

After so much intellectual weight and so many spiritual references have been tossed around, the final song (before the bland album-closing instrumental, 'Scandinavia') returns to nothing more than the individual. With Celtic choral sounds creating their own atmospheric mist, 'Across the Bridge Where Angels Dwell' simply advocates closing one's eyes 'in fields of wonder', dreaming of heaven and home. Both are waiting in that place where 'time is still'. And with all that has gone before, it's clear from *Beautiful Vision* that they are in fact the very same thing. Heaven is that place — that Celtic place — which all the while has been calling its prodigal sons home.

Cry for home (1975–1991)

INARTICULATE SPEECH OF THE HEART
(March 1983)

- Higher Than the World ▪ Connswater [instrumental]
- River of Time ▪ Celtic Swing [instrumental] ▪ Rave on, John Donne ▪ Inarticulate Speech of the Heart No. 1 [instrumental] ▪ Irish Heartbeat ▪ The Street Only Knew Your Name ▪ Cry For Home ▪ Inarticulate Speech of the Heart No. 2 ▪ September Night [instrumental]

Inarticulate Speech of the Heart may possess the most appalling title of any Van Morrison album but at a literal level it is an accurate description of the artist's work. Cutting through the technology of words in order to achieve a direct connection with the emotions is the fundamental task of many of Morrison's songs. As if to accentuate this, the album was originally intended to consist exclusively of instrumentals. Only four of these survived, and the lyrics in the formal 'songs' that replaced them are unusually explicit in their subject matter. The first half of the album is a spiritual state-of-the-union address, while the second is the most naked and ecstatic expression of love for origins that Morrison would ever record.

As on *Beautiful Vision*, there's a slick, commercial production and plenty of '80s-sounding synthesizers, but this time the recording sessions were spread across studios in London as well as California. Still, the music remains Irish to the core, with Davy Spillane's uillean pipes, Arty McGlynn's guitar and the sound of Celtic harmonies in the back-up vocals weaving in and out of the celebrations of identity.

The note of thanks to L. Ron Hubbard that appears on the cover is an anomaly. While Morrison had been interested in Scientology since first meeting and working with devotee Robin Williamson from the Incredible String Band, he was never a true believer. Certainly he attended meetings, and by one account proceeded to 'the fourth grade' of Scientology instruction, but a combination of his own independent nature and the Scientologists' demands for generous financial donations eventually sent him packing before he could join the ranks of the enlightened.

There is nothing in his work from this or any other period to suggest that Scientology had more influence on his modes of thought than other spiritual and religious movements. Indeed, on the shopping list of mystical cults name-checked on *Inarticulate Speech*'s 'Rave on, John Donne', Hubbard and Scientology don't even rate a mention among Theosophy, the Rosicrucians and the Hermetic Order of the Golden Dawn. Van never believed that humans were descended from aliens (as Scientologists do), but it's easy to understand his passing interest in a cult which considered that the key to enlightenment involves unlocking 'engrams' or 'mental knots' — those mechanical and illusory impediments to 'getting clear' at the mental and spiritual levels.

The real emotional force driving *Inarticulate Speech of the Heart* is what Morrison describes eponymously in 'Cry For Home'. Within the easy-listening New Age atmosphere of the album, these echoes of Irish instrumental and human voices permeate almost every track, as if tentacles are being stretched out across the Irish Sea in one direction, and the Atlantic Ocean in the other. In fact, the sequence of the tracks marks Van Morrison's journey homeward, beginning with spiritual ecstasy (in 'Higher Than the World'), then moving through a lengthy homage to literary and spiritual heroes who have lit the way (in 'Rave on, John Donne'), and eventually ending up back on the Belfast street corner with childhood friends Walter, John, Katie and Ron (in 'The Street Only Knew Your Name'). If *Inarticulate Speech of the Heart* is anything to go by, the cry for home and that coveted return to childhood has a more magnetic power on Morrison than any occult-based path to spiritual enlightenment. On every occasion, he would bypass the Scientology Centre on Tottenham Court Road in order — imaginatively — to get back to Hyndford Street in the 1950s.

Nevertheless, the album begins with the singer drifting up in the clouds, on 'Higher Than the World', the accompaniment moving in blocks of harmony as if 'the music of the spheres' mentioned in *Beautiful Vision* is now being made manifest. Not that Morrison was alone at this time in his penchant for meandering atmospherics — this was the era of Enya, Clannad and Windham Hill. What makes Morrison's take on the genre so distinctive, though, is that the slow-shifting harmonies of 'Higher Than the World' are punctuated by jazz guitar figures. And yet despite the initially ethereal quality of the vocals, as the tempo picks up in the middle of the song, the guttural voice so typical of this singer emerges involuntarily. As with his religion, Morrison is delving into the world of superior muzak without actually committing to it.

After the first of the Celtic instrumentals ('Connswater', whose vibrant folky rhythm also emerges from the shimmering harmonic mist), 'River of Time' has a thrilling power. It lunges forward repeatedly, each time leaning back on the deep bass notes to gain extra propulsion for the next surge. Lyrically, 'River of Time' is unexceptional — 'heart and soul, body and mind' are brought together on 'the river of time' — but on a musical level, it's a cracker, limited only by the laid-back, introspective vocal performance and the strange choice not to place it at the very beginning of the album.

'Celtic Swing', another instrumental (and, like 'Scandinavia' the previous year, a single in the UK), repeats the pattern of 'Connswater' by getting an Irish groove to emerge from vague New Age synthesizer meanderings. Soon, we're on to one of the definitive tracks of both this album and Morrison's work as a whole.

'Rave on, John Donne' apparently began in the studio as a 45-minute epic filling two complete 24-track tapes, frantic technicians trying to minimise the loss of material while the band played on through the tape change. The song is essentially narrated as poetry over by-now familiar synthesizer and jazz guitar figures — the same sound-world as 'Higher Than the World' — but now and again the passion of the vocals merges into actual singing, accentuated by Pee Wee Ellis's soprano sax embellishments. 'Rave on, John Donne' draws its distinctive (and easily parodied) character from the clashes of linguistic registers that see the modern rock slang 'rave on' thrown into stark relief against archaic literary phrases such as 'thy Holy fool' and 'O, what sweet wine we drinketh'.

Along with 'Summertime in England' and 'In the Days Before Rock 'n' Roll, this is the Van Morrison song that makes the most extravagant use of name-checks, with Walt Whitman, Omar Khayyam, Khalil Gibran and 'Mr Yeats' all

Cry for home (1975-1991)

getting a guernsey alongside the great lyric poet of the title (himself a cleric with an acute interest in sexual relations). Of these, however, the most relevant is perhaps Whitman, whose call to the future generations in 'Crossing Brooklyn Ferry' offers a parallel to the time-travel motif in 'Rave on, John Donne'. Morrison's song, which adds belated resonance to its predecessor 'River of Time', is about the transmission 'down through the weeks of ages' of the messages contained in the great literary writings and spiritual teachings. In his thesis, art ('words on printed page') survives the changing social fabric of the industrial revolution, empiricism and the atomic and nuclear age, and the coming and going of specialist religious fashions, and continues to provide inspiration to new generations and link the present with the past.

Morrison never advocates any of these schools of religious thought. As in many of the songs on *Beautiful Vision*, they are merely phases that the seeker encounters on his search, and all fall away as time exerts its force on them. In this, he is only a step away from his explicit proclamation three years later, 'No Guru, No Method, No Teacher'. And in spite of their diversity, the cults mentioned by Morrison are all concerned with finding an overriding unity within mystical experience. The Hermetic Order of the Golden Dawn (to which W.B. Yeats and occultist/mystic Aleister Crowley both belonged) sought coherence among the various specialist fields of the occult practices. The Rosicrucians ('the Holy Rosey Cross') believe that natural laws are interconnected in all their spiritual, physical, emotional and moral manifestations, while Theosophy also concerns itself with knowledge of the universe's inherent laws ('oneness of life').

In all of Morrison's musings on spirituality and philosophy, there is some sort of specific 'answer' to be found: the Holy Grail or Veedon Fleece of the searcher, or some similar key to unlocking the mysteries of the universe. But like a spiritual Sisyphus, whenever he ascends towards that one point of meaning, his guides let him down and he's back to the beginning again, left with the one thing that throughout it all orients his life. That one thing dominating all his work, and nowhere more so than in *Inarticulate Speech of the Heart*, is the celebration of home. Cults come and go, offering something of value here, an interesting idea there, but in the end, the enduring truth is of home. Which is why the great quest of 'Rave on, John Donne' is transformed — via the instrumental passage that is the album's title track — into 'Irish Heartbeat', with its assertion that the world cares 'nothing for/about your soul' in comparison with what you share 'with your own ones'. Out in this 'cold' world, you can never tell whether the stranger at your door is your best friend or your brother, so it's best not to stray too far from home. For a man who made his career doing the latter, this comes as some admission. The following songs only seek to confirm it.

'The Street Only Knew Your Name' says it all when the implicit answer to the singer's question in the lines 'Would you prefer all those castles in Spain / Or the view of your street from the window pane?' is that the latter is preferable. Life 'outside of the street' can never be complete. The 'centring' aesthetic that one day would reach its apotheosis with 'On Hyndford Street' is here established. The object of the previous dozen albums' quest is revealed as having been home all along, and the song ends in typical fashion with a

Cry for home (1975–1991)

name-check of Gene Vincent songs, being sung by Van and his childhood friends down on the street corner. How far we've travelled to end up back where it all began.

But there's more of the same to come. Indeed, the album's first single, 'Cry For Home' (which in the three words of its title might summarise Morrison's entire career), moves even further into the homecoming motif. On hearing this cry, the expatriates 'won't have to think at all'. The pull of origins transcends intellectual and spiritual searches. It is instantly recognisable, impossible to 'fake', and equally impossible to resist.

If this crucial philosophical revelation makes *Inarticulate Speech of the Heart* seem a less than convincing album in comparison with others by the same artist, it is surely because the definitive nature of its resolution means that its semantics are more constricted than on any other Van Morrison collection. Previous albums asked all the right questions, opening up the worlds of the songs to all manner of philosophical speculation and articulating both Morrison's and the listeners' human desire for knowledge and understanding; in *Inarticulate Speech of the Heart*, Morrison provides an answer. The trajectory of the album is towards resolution, limiting the scope of the enterprise as it proceeds on its inexorable journey towards meaning in childhood memory and a sense of belonging to a community. It's almost incongruous, therefore, that the album's final track, 'Inarticulate Speech of the Heart No. 2', repeats continually that 'I'm a soul in wonder'. On any other Van Morrison album, this would be very true, but here the statement has never seemed less accurate.

A working man in his prime

For one of the few times in his career to that point, *Inarticulate Speech of the Heart* answered all the questions that were being asked, and the Morrison soul — if only temporarily — was in wonder no more. He'd come home and everything made sense again. And that sense was of wonder.

A SENSE OF WONDER
(December 1984)

■ *Tore Down à la Rimbaud* ■ *Ancient of Days* ■ *Evening Meditation* [instrumental] ■ *The Master's Eyes* ■ *What Would I Do* ■ *A Sense of Wonder* ■ *Boffyflow and Spike* [instrumental] ■ *If You Only Knew* ■ *Let the Slave* (incorporating *The Price of Experience*) ■ *A New Kind of Man*

The pattern of the mid 1970s was repeated in the mid 1980s. Just as the 'return to home' of *Veedon Fleece* in 1974 had precipitated a crisis of identity and writer's block, so too the even more explicit celebration of home in *Inarticulate Speech of the Heart* in 1983 caused Van Morrison to run out of questions to ask. The creative wasteland returned and it would be close to two years before his next collection appeared — an unthinkably long wait at any time in the singer's career apart from the lost years of 1975–76.

For Morrison's fans, the gap was filled by the release of his second live album, concert appearances with both the recently re-formed Band and Bob Dylan (separately this time), and further touring — including his only, unsatisfactory visit to Australia. If nothing else, *Live at the Grand Opera House,*

Cry for home (1975–1991)

Belfast served as a showcase for Morrison's outstanding band, which, like the legendary Caledonia Soul Orchestra, took a number of years to morph its way into its definitive line-up of Chris Michie (lead guitar), John Allair (keyboards), Pee Wee Ellis (saxophone and flute, and one of Van's great musical arrangers), Mark Isham (trumpet and keyboards, soon to depart for a career as a film composer in Hollywood), David Hayes (dependable as ever on bass), Peter van Hooke and Tom Donlinger (both playing drums), and Katie Kissoon, Bianca Thornton and Carol Kenyon (his trio of backing vocalists).

When at last he did release a new studio album — now as an international Mercury artist for the first time — its opening track not only lamented, chorus by chorus, 'I wish my message [/purpose/writing] would come', but more significantly its origins dated back to those other 'fallow' creative years around 1975. As in this song, 'Tore Down à la Rimbaud', Morrison's fourteenth album finds the singer looking for inspiration in the work of the great poets. Not so much a homage piece as a vaguely desperate plea for a creative direction, *A Sense of Wonder* includes only five original full songs, a couple of instrumentals, a setting by others of William Blake's poetry, and two standards, penned by musical heroes Ray Charles and Mose Allison.

Still, the album has more to recommend it than its potential counterpart, *A Period of Transition*. Unlike the sound-world of that 1977 drought-breaker, the obsession with poetry was an essential ingredient of the singer's personality, and the incidental collaboration with Irish folk-rock band Moving Hearts sowed aesthetic seeds that would germinate with outstanding success in future work. *A Sense of Wonder*, in other words, was also a period of transition, but this time it led somewhere important.

Paradoxically, given that it's a song about the absence of creative inspiration, 'Tore Down à la Rimbaud' makes for a lively opening track, Morrison sounding engaged and energetic. The French symbolist Arthur Rimbaud is an appropriate exemplar of the concerns expressed in the song, having achieved youthful success before being driven into silence by the hammering that his precocious teenage poetry received from the critics. The song is a manifesto and a celebration of all the things that creative art gives its listeners — knowledge of self, visions, nightmares, light at the end of a tunnel, days of deep devotion, and different shapes, colours and roads leading out of the dark night of the soul. Just like Walt Whitman before him, Van Morrison loves this catalogue technique, and sometimes it seems as if his songs grow out of dot points listing sources of inspiration. These catalogued functions of great art begin *A Sense of Wonder*, and the album's title track ends with another list, but this time of favourite childhood foodstuffs. 'Ancient of Days' also has a catalogue technique, built around the phrases 'Saw you shining[/standing/stirring/moving]', with the title appended after each verse. The Ancient of Days in question derives both from the Bible and also from the title of a William Blake illustration, but nothing is made of the allusion in the song; it's simply another name-check used for its evocative power rather than illustrating or exemplifying some kind of meaning. Nevertheless, the 'ancient of days' mentioned in Psalm 69 does have some connection with Morrison's work as a whole. In its biblical meaning, the Ancient of Days is the face that the Lord shines down on the righteous when the mood so strikes him, and the believer who looks up towards the face is referred to as 'the impatient one'. In 'Dweller on the Threshold' a couple of years earlier, Van had characterised himself as that impatient spiritual searcher, tired of waiting for the moment of enlightenment. The buoyant 'Ancient of Days' recreates the ebullient musical mood of that earlier song, and perhaps somewhere deep down in Morrison's subconscious, it also picks up on the spiritual impatience of the protagonist. Certainly, the song's quest for a dominant spiritual guru feeds into the album's next song.

Following the oddly intense wordless vocal of 'Evening Meditation', 'The Master's Eyes' is one of Morrison's most musically poignant numbers, part Irish Protestant hymn and part African–American spiritual, but the identity of the Master in question is never revealed. It could be a guru or God himself, or it could be a vision (which is certainly the view of Morrison's musician-colleague Clive Culbertson, who maintains that it was *his* vision, which he had narrated to Van!). The vital line is 'And my questions all were answered', just as they had been on *Inarticulate Speech of the Heart*. What the answer is, we never learn, except that it comes in the form of light shining from the Master's eyes, but such a revelation leads to an artistic impasse: we, the listeners, neither share in the experience nor have any understanding of what it might actually be. In fact, both 'Ancient of Days' and 'The Master's Eyes' are notable for their sound more than their sense. Both refer to spiritual topics without elucidating them in any way — two of the few occasions in his career when the constant criticisms that Morrison's 'intellectual' references are superficial might perhaps be justified. For all the sense that the two songs make, they might as well bear the titles 'Be-bop' and 'A-lula'. By the time of his next album release, the search for a guru that both tracks describe would be cast aside without a second thought.

Much more depth is revealed in the title track, which follows after the dreamy, reverential version of Ray Charles's 'What Would I Do'. 'A Sense of Wonder' was the first single off the album ('Tore Down à la Rimbaud' followed early in the new year) and it's a hypnotic recounting of those childhood 'days of blooming wonder', with Van out walking in his greatcoat through the inevitable falling autumn leaves, over Newtonards and Comba, Gransha and the Ballystockart Road. But even here, in such familiar Morrison territory, there remains the problem of writer's block. It's 'easy' to write about the beauty of autumn, the song says, but what about the winter of discontent during the months of January and February? They are 'a very different thing'. Morrison resolves the dilemma by ignoring it, going on to list various Belfast street scenes from his youth. Again, the song sounds beautiful, but there's only the usual nostalgic catalogue to keep its lyrics going.

Van was waiting for his next big idea to come, and it would do so with extraordinary power in time for the following album. But in the meantime, there was a second side of an album to fill. He filled the empty space firstly with a run-through of Mose Allison's 'If You Only Knew', and then through the agency of poet Adrian Mitchell and composer/arranger Mike Westbrook.

Cry for home (1975–1991)

That duo's adaptation of Blake's 'The Price of Experience', titled 'Let the Slave', furnished Morrison with the most political and revolutionary text that he would offer up on any album. A companion piece to 'Let the Slave' would have been William Mathieu's setting of W.B. Yeats's 'Crazy Jane on God' (indeed, it was, on early promotional copies of *A Sense of Wonder*), another spiritual meditation from a mystically inclined poetic champion. The Yeats estate refused permission for the text to appear in a non-classical setting, however, and the track was withdrawn before the album's commercial release. (It finally appeared on *The Philosopher's Stone* in June 1998, by which time Yeats's words were out of copyright.)

The only remaining Morrison originals on the album are the instrumental 'Boffyflow and Spike' — two characters who also make appearances in the title song and in Morrison's whimsical liner notes — and the song 'A New Kind of Man', whose title is taken from a William Blake biography. This track finds Morrison lifting up his eyes towards the mountain-top, trying to gain some perspective on the 'trials' that he has undergone and hoping that they 'have not been in vain'. Just as in 'The Master's Eyes', there's a light shining ahead and he's sure that it's 'part of a plan', but the specifics once more are left vague.

While such clichés litter this bits-and-pieces album of attractive-sounding quests for inspiration, there really was a light shining just up ahead. After another long gap by Van Morrison's standards — over eighteen months — by which time the 23-year-old singer of *Astral Weeks* would have passed the milestone age of forty, a new album arrived, and it was a masterpiece.

A working man in his prime

NO GURU, NO METHOD, NO TEACHER
(July 1986)

- *Got to Go Back* - *Oh the Warm Feeling* - *Foreign Window* - *A Town Called Paradise* - *In the Garden* - *Tir Na Nog* - *Here Comes the Knight* - *Thanks for the Information* - *One Irish Rover* - *Ivory Tower*

On *Into the Music*, Van Morrison had introduced the concept of music as a healing force, a subject that he discussed regularly with colleagues like Robin Williamson, Clive Culbertson, and Derek Bell from the Chieftains. By 1986, when *No Guru, No Method, No Teacher* was released, the idea that music could not just heal but also open other mental and spiritual horizons had become a fascination that not only influenced the music and lyrics, but also had extra-curricular appeal.

Around this time, Morrison teamed up with the Wrekin Trust, whose brief was to awaken the vision of the spiritual nature of man and the universe. Indeed, in the year after *No Guru* appeared, Morrison in partnership with the trust organised a three-day conference at Loughborough University devoted to an exploration of how the power of music could change consciousness. But the signs of this more conscious and sophisticated approach to the concept of music therapy were already there for all to see in *No Guru*, an album so cogent, organic and so germane to Van Morrison's art that its themes (of which healing was a crucial one) and sublime music make it arguably the signature recording of the artist's career.

Clearly, the title alone is a manifesto. After years of public speculation about Morrison's religious beliefs, and his references to the likes of L. Ron Hubbard, Rosicrucianism, the Jehovah's Witnesses, Meher Baba, Krishnamurti and various other spiritual 'masters', at last Morrison came right out and said it. There was no intermediary between him and his God — no quasi-divine teacher, no formalised system of belief or worship, and no single instructor in the ways of faith.

Not that it's an anti-religious album. On the contrary, *No Guru, No Method, No Teacher* is as 'Christian' in its sentiments as anything he ever recorded, but the Christianity on display is not the formal going-to-church-on-Sunday type. Instead, it concerns itself with the direct, unmediated apprehension of and communion with God. More importantly, the faith so amply displayed on the album operates within a whole host of other Morrison themes, each balanced against the other to create a complete world view.

Fittingly for an album that broke such new ground in his recent work, the recording sessions saw some major changes in Morrison's tight circle of musicians. Gone now were Allair, Ellis, van Hooke and Donlinger, their places at Sausalito and London's Townhouse Studios filled with a combination of old hands and those who would make just this single-album contribution. In a move that saw almost half of the Caledonia Soul Orchestra reunited, Jeff Labes returned on keyboards (having last worked with Van on some arrangements for *Common One*), John Platania joined Chris Michie on lead guitar, and cellist Terry Adams arranged the strings; bass player David Hayes had rarely left the Ulsterman's employ, of course. But *No Guru, No Method, No Teacher* would be no blast from the past.

A working man in his prime

Musically, it begins with the feel of a boat bobbing on the ocean — a momentary drum flourish, deep bass throbbing, and Kate St John's oboe drifting sublimely over the top. This intro to 'Got to Go Back' is like Walt Whitman's 'Out of the Cradle Endlessly Rocking' transformed into musical form. And the topic? It's the familiar homecoming — not just for the sake of re-establishing identity but more urgently 'for the healing'. Indeed, the opening verse of 'Got to Go Back' is an explication of the themes and ideas that had sustained Morrison's career, but which here are stated so clearly that they comprise a definitive statement.

The lyrics begin with the nostalgic Van singing in unusually hushed and awed tones about being a schoolboy back in Orangefield, looking out the window of his classroom and dreaming, before going home to be inspired by the music of Ray Charles. The message he hears from the great blind seer is about belief in the soul, the very thought of which lifts him up and leads him to meditation and contemplation. There, in the first minute of Van Morrison's masterpiece, lies the essence of his art. The chorus argues that a return to that world is essential 'for the healing' and to 'go on with the dreaming'.

By the second verse, the meditation class has begun, with the lyrics instructing the breath to go right down into the stomach and then to be exhaled in 'radiance'. With these techniques of transcendental meditation established, Swami Van begins to muse on his own career, and how in particular he's been 'living in a foreign country that operates along completely different lines' from those with which he grew up. It's a theme of expatriation that dates back to *Astral Weeks*, but which here and in 'Foreign Window' receives its most extended and moving analysis.

Morrison himself is moved by the fact that he's come home after all those years. He asks to be kept away from strong liquor and anything sentimental because they'll just make him cry. Here, in this sublime opening, the old curmudgeon reveals the softie within. He weeps the tears of the returned Danny Boy, peeling off the foreign culture in a revelation of the true religion within him — the love of Ireland and home, and music. There *is* actually a kind of guru, there is a method and an inanimate teacher: it's called home. And never did a man sound as happy and relieved to be there as Van Morrison at the start of this sublime album. Released in the UK as the second single off *No Guru*, 'Got to Go Back' is far more representative of its parent album's strengths than the first choice, the terse 'Ivory Tower'.

The mood is maintained in the second song, appropriately titled 'Oh the Warm Feeling'. Uncomplicated in its lyrics (it simply speaks of gladness at being with another), 'Oh the Warm Feeling' nevertheless introduces a crucial theme of the album as a whole. Or rather, it offers an intersection of various themes. As he sits beside his lover, the protagonist is 'filled . . . with religion'. Throughout this album, and like *Beautiful Vision*, a parallel is established between sexual love and spiritual enlightenment, as if each song sits at that crossroads where the carnal and the cosmic meet. More than that, the romantic concept of the solitary spiritual searcher is abandoned; instead, moments of revelation are communal. It's two people helping each other along the road to heaven, with Morrison genuinely feeling the emotion of another in a way in which he hadn't done since the final tracks of *Veedon Fleece* (significantly, another 'homecoming' album). Love leads to spiritual awakening, and revelation is something that the lovers can experience together, one helping the other, showing the way, offering encouragement, and whispering tales of paradise just ahead. For this reason alone, *No Guru* lays some claim to being Morrison's greatest collection of love songs. But it is much else besides.

In a television documentary in which Morrison plays 'Foreign Window' with a bewildered Bob Dylan sitting beside him in front of the Acropolis in Athens, the singer himself admits that he has no idea what the album's third track means. From the lyrics, we gather he's watching someone from a foreign window who's 'bearing down the sufferin' road'. In fact, the meaning of this densely structured song seems clear enough. From an alien perspective, he is observing a fellow spiritual searcher — referred to in the second person throughout, but let's presume the subject is female, his lover — suffering under her 'burden' as she seeks out 'the palace of the Lord'. Again, in this image the pursuit of enlightenment is the source of suffering and pain — not just joy or ecstasy.

A passing reference to Whitman ('When the lilacs were in bloom') leads into another ambiguous verse, in which the searcher is on the sofa with the sun shining through, and she's going through her prayers 'That the masters had instilled' in her. Even such a positive image reminds us of Lord Byron's love of despair: the loss of hope and the experience of suffering accompany any spiritual or artistic venture. But, as the bridge insists, if we 'get it right', we 'don't have to come back again' — a rare Morrison reference to reincarnation, it

Cry for home (1975–1991)

seems. More pertinent to this album, however, are lines three and four of the same bridge: 'And if you get it right this time / There's no need to explain'. That's Van Morrison's idea of heaven: where words simply fall away, irrelevant because a direct connection with the Platonic ideal (or God) has been established. But in the meantime, like John Bunyan's Pilgrim and the Everyman of the medieval miracle plays, we're still searching in a foreign country, trying to find our way back home. That home is, in itself, a spiritual state.

In the third verse of 'Foreign Window', Morrison introduces a ploy, sustained elsewhere in the album, where he sings about someone else but his writing is blatantly autobiographical. In this first instance, the 'you' in question is 'singing about Rimbaud', which, of course, Morrison himself had done on his previous album. And as the song proceeds, and he offers his lover protection 'against the loneliness of the crowd', it becomes clear that we're hearing about *his* journey too, not just hers. In the meantime, everyone's giving her religion and the ceremonies of 'breaking bread and drinking wine' continue, but the real hope for enlightenment comes when the searcher lies out 'on the green hills, just like when you were a child'.

The message is an anti-material one. The rituals and the alienation of social organisation are not paths to the truth. In the palace of the Lord, the searcher sleeps 'on a pallet on the floor', and all the glamour and bustle and possessions of the day-to-day world are transcended — but with no guaranteed result — in the direct, unmediated encounter with God. To get back home (again, heaven and home are the one thing), you have to renounce the demands placed on you by the crowd. Were you a popular singer, for instance, this might well mean abandoning the enhanced commercial prospects of the American record industry for a simpler life in Ireland.

The shared experience between two spiritual searchers continues in the up-tempo, *Astral Weeks*-like 'A Town Called Paradise', with its imagery of two people climbing a mountainside, and in subsequent verses riding both the musical groove and the 'ancient highway' together. It begins, though, a world away, in the culture of complaint — that unfortunate thematic preoccupation that would jeopardise Morrison's songwriting reputation in the 1990s. Fortunately here, the opening complaints about people ripping off his songs are dropped as soon as they appear, and the song proceeds with the uplifting refrain that despite all these frustrations, 'All that matters is my relationship to you'. Whether the song is addressed to girlfriend Ulla Munch (whom colleagues all attest had a positive influence on Van Morrison's personality around this time) or a more generalised or mythical lover, the song restates the album's ongoing theme, that sexual love and spiritual enlightenment go hand in hand. The destination is a town called Paradise and the means to get there are the lover, the car and a reverence for the past. And how do we know when we get there? Martin Drover's muted trumpet peels out a descant like Sunday church bells and the song fades out with the service beckoning . . .

The masterly 'In the Garden' begins with an explicitly erotic image: a vision of woman standing in a garden 'wet with rain'. After a summer shower, she's crying and the singer too is feeling a 'great sadness'. Presumably this same suffering woman was the protagonist of 'Foreign Window'. Here, though, there is a dramatic transformation between her 'bearing down the sufferin' road' in the first verse and how she appears in the second. When she returns to the garden for that second appearance, she has become radiant ('a creature all in rapture') and she has found the 'keys' to her soul — which she is not afraid to open for the admiring Van. And as we teeter on that precipice between erotic and spiritual ecstasy, the light of God shines down on her face. The colour of the radiance is violet, as is the album cover, as is holiness in Yeats's 'Oil and Blood', and as is the homeward journey in T.S. Eliot's 'The Waste Land'. And she feels the summer breeze on her as she sits beside her father and mother. She's come home. Or rather, Van Morrison has come home, for again, the hushed and awestruck tones of the vocals indicate that this glorious, most personal song is as much about the singer as the subject. (Indeed, is the reference to 'violet colour' intended as an act of homage to his own mother, Violet?)

And once home, the radiant one goes into the familiar Morrison trance and the 'childlike vision' emerges again to the accompaniment of Sunday church bells. At that point, the Veedon Fleece (or Holy Grail) shows itself, but not in the anticipated form of divine inspiration or even backstreet jellyroll. Rather, the perfect spiritual state turns out to be eternal youth — a Morrison theme revealed for the first time here and destined to be worked over again on subsequent albums.

This revelation of eternal summer and youth that never ages throws the singer's earlier work into starker relief. In his perfect world, the past furnishes the present, indeed *is* the present, and as in 'Sweet Thing' from so many years earlier, we will 'never grow so old again'. This fascination with youth may explain why, after 'T.B. Sheets' in 1967, nobody ever dies in a Van Morrison song. The old people are 'ancients' who live on, either as spiritual powers or — in the case of poets and singers — as ongoing inspirations. Ray Charles, for instance, may be 'shot down' but he still 'got up to do his best'. In many ways, it's Wordsworth's 'Intimations of Immortality' transformed into the modern era.

Eternal youth now established, the love object of 'In the Garden' is 'born again', and as the singer touches her cheeks 'so lightly', these two (literal) soul-mates feel the presence of Christ in their hearts. Even though the church that they both love so much is close enough to hear, they're still outside in nature, and the revelation and transformation has occurred there, close by but beyond the four walls of organised religion. The presence of Christ is immediate, intuited by them in the natural environment without the interception of the preacher or the guru or society at large. It's just them, nature and the Father, himself transformed from the literal father of the 'homecoming verse' to the spiritual father — another equation between home and heaven.

As the song descends to almost nothing, with just acoustic guitar accompanying Van's whispers, then brushes and the odd bass note, the Father is joined by the Son and the Holy Ghost. The revelation occurs with this direct communion with the Holy Trinity, and the journey towards silence and meditation reaches the limit of popular recorded music's ability to convey it.

Although here the song simply peters out, live versions of 'In the Garden' include a resurrection of the tempo and the band, with a rousing chorus of the line 'No guru, no method, no teacher' ringing out as Van departs the stage. In concert, it's filled with revivalist fervour, the congregation singing their hearts out in joy and ecstasy, but in the concert hall rather than the church. This spiritual triumph effectively summarises Morrison's art, and the song itself reveals a magical, intensely beautiful vision of a perfect world whose radiance and charm are impossible to resist.

Several of the ideas contained in the album's first half are picked up again in 'Tir Na Nog', the first Van Morrison song ever to feature a Gaelic title. For the Celts, Tir Na Nog is a mythical land of eternal youth; in Morrison's narrative, again, the lovers are on their way there. As in 'A Town Called Paradise', the journey goes up a mountain-side, and as in 'In the Garden', it passes by a church — named explicitly (also for the first time in Morrison's work) as the Church of Ireland — where the pilgrims stop to pray. And as the lovers continue to be enraptured by the silence, it seems that the travelling companion is in fact not just a lover but a 'long-lost friend . . . from another lifetime'.

We're in the deathless world of eternity and reincarnation, and the phrases chosen to depict the environment are equally reincarnated from Morrison's earlier, and future, writings: it's a 'golden autumn day', the garden again is 'wet with rain', and there's the obligatory 'cool, clear crystal stream'. Once more, this is Blake's New Jerusalem as a storm rages outside, and, in an echo from *Astral Weeks*, while Van meditates, his lover kisses his eyes. As is so often the way, these Morrison clichés only serve a greater purpose, which in this case is to ask: 'How can we not be attached? After all, we're only human.' The attachment in question is not to God (let alone guru or method) but to other human beings.

In an extraordinarily revealing moment, Morrison appears to be stating that spiritual experience and the journey towards enlightenment is unappetising without his great love beside him. And great love is surely what the entire album is about. The resolution comes not in spiritual nirvana — because as the lyrics state, there is no way back from that — but in acknowledgement that ultimate meaning exists in the love between two people. Spirituality remains a vital search but, on this album at least, it is valuable only if accompanied by a revered companion. The gurus and the methods have to make way for a lover. And it's in this way that *No Guru, No Method, No Teacher* is simultaneously Van Morrison's greatest 'philosophical journey' and his greatest album of love songs.

Back in the land of eternal youth, 'Tir Na Nog' drifts off with Morrison keening vigorously in the Irish voice of the ages, eternal and assured at last of his place within the mystical kingdom of eternal youth. Now, with all the temporal boundaries of chronology removed, Morrison's mind is free to wander.

In a dubious pun on the title of one of Them's hits, 'Here Comes the Knight' transports us back into a feudal world, where quotations from Yeats are thrown together in a curious medieval stew. Echoing Arthurian legend, there are horsemen riding by, but their message (adapted from Yeats's epitaph to 'Under Ben Bulben') is that a 'cold eye' should be kept on life and death alike, and that truth to self is the ultimate spiritual achievement. The gist of the song's evocation of courtly love is again eternal — 'this love will surely last forever [/always]' — but again the culture of complaint raises its ugly head. We hear that Van has been accused of 'truth and alchemy' — in other words, he's been praised and criticised — and there are people who 'don't want this love to last'. Once more, though, with the vile crowd clamouring for 'a demonstration' from Van the Man, the matter is resolved in love: all that ultimately matters (although this time it is not stated) is 'my relationship to you'.

The album never really loses its momentum, but neither do the final three tracks particularly add to the uplifting mood. In fact, 'Thanks for the Information' risks bringing it all crashing down with its series of sarcastic complaints about people always giving and getting the wrong information. The song is built of clichés and commonplaces ('Never give a sucker an even break', 'I should look before I leap', etc.). It also invokes the New Testament reference (Matthew 19:30) once employed by Dylan (in 'The Times They Are A-Changin''') to the first being last and the last first. The crucial message of 'Thanks for the Information', however, is one of frustration, not just with people offering advice, but more particularly with the spiritual search itself. There are always obstacles in the way, and never more so than when the searcher is 'breaking through to a new level of consciousness'. Again, the search for meaning is continually frustrated; it's 'two steps forward' and 'three back', and 'what you gain on the hobbyhorse you lose on the swing'. For this most truculent of songwriters, even the quests for transcendence that have sustained his career remain a big pain in the arse.

A working man in his prime

The album is winding down now and while the gentle 'One Irish Rover' is clearly intended as another autobiography, it doesn't rise much beyond a request for an Irish story, some facts, and the question of whether the respondent can 'see the light'. The lover now is far away, gone astray like a ship out on the sea. The majestic homecoming of the album's first half might never have happened; the mystical quest has descended into mere repetition.

This impression is only exacerbated on the final track, 'Ivory Tower'. Abandoning all sense of mysticism in favour of a straight r&b bitch session, Morrison invites his critics to come down from their lofty place of judgement to spend a moment in his shoes. They're people who offer opinions on things they 'know nothing about' and have no idea of the price Van has to pay to do the things he does. Enough said. It's hard to inspire others while whingeing, but at least the buoyant vocal suggests that Van was managing to interest himself in his latest gripe, and the fleeting reference to 'glamour' indicates that Alice Bailey still had an influence.

No Guru, No Method, No Teacher, which ascends closer to heaven than anything Morrison had previously achieved, concludes with graceless complaints. Yet as this crowning achievement of his career mentions elsewhere, no matter how much divine inspiration may touch us, 'we're only human'. It would be unrealistic to expect that an album that makes such important aesthetic strides towards eternity should remain untouched by the grubby marks of the truculent and embittered human hands that created it.

Cry for home (1975–1991)

POETIC CHAMPIONS COMPOSE
(September 1987)

■ *Spanish Steps [instrumental]* ■ *The Mystery* ■ *Queen of the Slipstream* ■ *I Forgot that Love Existed* ■ *Sometimes I Feel Like a Motherless Child* ■ *Celtic Excavation [instrumental]* ■ *Someone Like You* ■ *Alan Watts Blues* ■ *Give Me My Rapture* ■ *Did Ye Get Healed?* ■ *Allow Me [instrumental]*

How does one follow a masterpiece? Van Morrison's initial reaction was to practise his saxophone, engage new musicians, move to a new studio in England's West Country, and record an album of instrumentals. But after three tracks of ambient sax solos over slow-moving 'Celtic' accompaniments, the idea was ditched (as it had been on *Inarticulate Speech of the Heart*), and the players assembled at Bath's Wool Hall Studios were left to jam their way into another song-based album. While only trumpeter Martin Drover and guitarist Mick Cox had appeared on previous Morrison albums (the latter way back on *Common One*), three of these new musicians would prove to be mainstays of Morrison's sessions over the next few years: keyboard player Neil Drinkwater, bassist Steve Pearce and orchestral arranger Fiachra Trench.

Poetic Champions Compose has become one of the most hotly debated works of Morrison's career, dividing critics and biographers in their opinions of its quality. Patrick Humphries found 'little to excite or inspire', reasoning that 'we had all been down this well-trodden road just a few too many times before', while John Collis considered it to be one of Van's 'less inspired' efforts. Brian Hinton believed it was his 'third masterpiece on a roll', however, and Clinton Heylin calls it 'everything that *Inarticulate Speech of the Heart* had attempted to be — yearning, beguiling, musically adventurous, even tender on occasions'.

The contradictory critical responses might have been prompted by Morrison's perceived arrogance in turning the spiritual journey of *No Guru, No Method, No Teacher* into a series of declarations about the ways to achieve enlightenment. In a transition filled with artistic risk, on *Poetic Champions Compose* the troubled searcher becomes the spiritual guide himself. And as one might have expected, he proves to be something of a harsh master, in the very first song telling his pupils, 'Trust what I say and do as you're told'. Musically, however, the album holds its own with its predecessor, not least because of the outstanding production quality and musicianship. Van even manages to get his saxophone playing up to a reasonable standard. In the old LP format, both sides opened with instrumentals ('Spanish Steps' and the interestingly titled 'Celtic Excavation') and the second side closed with one also ('Allow Me') — the only indication of Morrison's original intentions.

'The Mystery', which opens the formal eight-song component of the album, picks up on *No Guru*'s reference to alchemy. If you wish to penetrate the mystery, it seems, you must 'open up your heart' and listen to Van the Master, and then 'all your dirt will turn into gold'. The first of these lines represents the start of the album's catalogue of Morrison clichés and dates back to its extended treatment on *Common One*, while the idea of transforming dirt is an early reference

Cry for home (1975–1991)

to the Philosopher's Stone, the base metal that, via the alchemical process, turns into gold.

As his previous albums demonstrated, travelling the 'mystic road' to spiritual riches is difficult and requires 'some faith to carry on'. In an aural pun, Morrison sings that you have to open up your heart 'to the sun', only for it to resolve into the Son, and the realisation that the song bears an explicitly Christian message. Once that particular faith is established, the next step is to 'dance and sing', 'be alive', 'be joyous and give thanks' — all those things that were happening on *Wavelength* with the Jehovah's Witnesses 'down at the Kingdom Hall'. No doubt about it, during Morrison's intermittent though career-long flirtations with Christianity, whenever he goes to worship he boogies and swings with the best of them, a legacy no doubt of a childhood that mixed fleeting participation in a revivalist sect with the fervour of a gospel record collector. On this particular track, everyone's heading in the same direction. The light of ancient Greece points towards 'the One', while Morrison himself (again with a companion) is in reach 'of the sun [/Son]'.

The idea of mystery is picked up again in 'Queen of the Slipstream', in the form of a secret that the lover must not share, and the gold of the previous track also appears, laid (along with silver) at the lover's feet. The title naturally recalls the opening line of *Astral Weeks* ('If I ventured in the slipstream'). While no one has ever truly penetrated the mystery of the said 'slipstream', it seems to serve two functions. On one hand, the slipstream is the private place where the dreamer establishes his own identity within a massive, constantly changing universe. It's that little tributary of the river where unique individual experience feeds into a greater whole, a pool of consciousness perhaps. As such, it is the fluvial equivalent of that other common Morrison term, 'backstreet'. On the other hand, in physics a slipstream is also that momentum gained through the lodgement of an object in the wake of forward propulsion. And as any competitive road cyclist knows, the quickest way to a destination is to share in the force of a group travelling in a particular direction. One rides with the power and submits any personal identity to the momentum generated by the pack. In 'the slipstream', then, the spiritual searcher is on the fast-track to the desired end — an idea surely irresistible to Morrison in his impatient quest for spiritual answers.

If these interpretations are correct, the 'queen' in question is another of those companions who in *No Guru* and elsewhere accompany the pilgrim Morrison on his quest. And she's been through a lot just to get to this point, having crossed many rivers, drunk from the fountain of innocence (a neat combination of Blake's innocence and Morrison's own recent fascination with the fountain of youth) and experienced the long, cold wintry years. But the secret world that is revealed to these frequently separated lovers — 'far away across the sea', similar to the description in the previous album's 'Irish Rover' — is not now Christian so much as it is literary. This 'dream' is of a place where the 'poetic champions compose'.

Presumably, the face of the Ancient of Days reveals itself here in the likeness of William Blake. But even at this anticipated moment of revelation, Van the Master is confident enough to announce that she'll choose him instead. Unspeakably vain on one literal level, in terms of Morrison's writing as a whole it is the obverse of *No Guru*'s line 'All that matters is my relationship to you'. Spiritual enlightenment is all well and good, but it's worthless unless aligned with genuine human emotion. As such, 'Queen of the Slipstream', with its distinctive use of what sounds like a Celtic harp, could have sat comfortably within the philosophical thesis of the previous album.

The same argument is reiterated on the next track, 'I Forgot that Love Existed', in which the singer notes that Socrates and Plato (the second reference in three songs to ancient Greece) praised love 'to the skies'. The desire expressed here is to reverse the mental and emotional senses, so that the heart can do the thinking and the head can begin to feel, revealing a new vision of the world and a more acute sense of reality. More particularly, the song simply repeats the philosophical conclusion of *No Guru* — that love is the highest spiritual power and the ultimate destination of any philosophical search. If the answer is disappointing, it's simply because the question is always rich semantically, and the answer inevitably closes off possibilities in the listener's imagination. Worse than that, the argument summarised by the Beatles as 'All you need is love' is hardly original.

'Sometimes I Feel Like a Motherless Child' is the American spiritual that Van Morrison was bound to record, its poignant desire for home fuelling so much of his own writing over the years. And the version recorded here, with its punchy bass line, itchy-feet guitar licks and heartfelt vocals, takes it way beyond its origins while still remaining true to the essential message. Amid its sense of abandonment and desire for repatriation, Morrison proved his natural gifts as a folksinger, paving the way (via an American tradition) to the *Irish Heartbeat* sessions of the following year.

Poetic Champions Compose marks Van Morrison's move into so-called 'easy-listening' music suitable for an older demographic. While there are plenty of dreamy New Age instrumentals from earlier albums that fit the forget-your-troubles format — and the three wordless pieces on *Poetic Champions* add to that tally — the songs themselves had tended to shy away from muzak and the sounds of the retirement village. All that changed, however with, 'Someone Like You', which is a direct precursor to the old-age wallpaper music of 'Have I Told You Lately' that would emerge within two years. Unsurprisingly, it was one of three tracks from this collection that were selected as singles in the UK (the others being 'Did Ye Get Healed?' and 'Queen of the Slipstream').

With its dreamy melody, saccharine banality and Zimmer-frame pace, 'Someone Like You' could represent the nadir of a creative talent that started so long ago with the screaming leprechaun antics of Them. But the song maintains some morbid interest simply because it begins to roll out one Morrison cliché after another. In order, Van has been 'searching a long time', 'travelling all around the world', 'travellin' a hard road', 'carryin' a heavy load', 'waiting for the light to come shining through', 'doin' some soul searching', going 'up and down the highway', 'in all kinds of foreign lands', and so on. In *No Guru*'s 'Thanks for the Information', he made a virtue of quoting other people's clichés. Here he makes the mistake of doing the same with his own.

Much more interesting is 'Alan Watts Blues', which is not blues at all, more like a shuffle. Alan Watts, whom Morrison knew personally, was a member of the Beat generation, the author of texts on Eastern mysticism, and an acknowledged authority on Zen Buddhism until his death in 1973. An important work of his was *Cloud Hidden, Whereabouts Unknown: A Mountain Journal*, inspired by a T'ang Dynasty Chinese poem that, in its original form, reads: 'I asked the boy beneath the pines / He said, "The master's gone alone / Herb-picking somewhere on the mount, / Cloud hidden, whereabouts unknown."'

The phrase 'Cloud hidden, whereabouts unknown' recurs throughout the song as Morrison plans to get himself 'out of the rat-race' and enjoy some time with his 'quiet friend'. In fact, like his quiet friend Watts, he's going up to the mountain-top once more, in solitude, to watch the fog roll in, in the hope that it will do him 'some good' and allow him to escape (in a nice mix of rodent metaphors) 'the ways of mice and men'. While the principles of Zen Buddhism have been implicit in so much of Morrison's work, especially in the journeys towards silence and meditation, this latest trek up the mountain-side and the explicit invocation of Alan Watts indicated a growing fascination with the kind of Zen thoughts that would soon result in speculation about the sound of one hand clapping.

Unlike previous Morrison songs, the journey of 'Alan Watts Blues' ends back down at the bottom. The searcher has been up the mountain and returned; now with his car motor running, he is preparing to return to civilisation. He knows he'll be back at the mountain sometime later, but for the moment, the resolution is an abandonment of the search. There's nothing to suggest disillusionment at the spiritual level, but the prosaic 'waiting in a clearing' while he sits in his car certainly indicates fatigue on the part of the lyricist.

Evidently, when the searcher drives off from the mountain retreat, he heads to a Christian church. 'Give Me My Rapture' begins with the singer musing on the strange things that happen every day and how they fill him with wonder. In a return to the music of the spheres motif, he hears music playing above his head and he's transported into rapture, leading immediately to a contemplation of divinity and the desire to 'sing all day'. Again, it's that joyous Christianity that provides the staying power to overcome the ubiquitous 'dark night of the soul' and fuels the boundless energy of the believer. The third verse opens up a direct plea bargain with the Lord to be worthy and to receive blessings 'into my life'. It's Van teaching us, and himself, how to pray and to 'purify my words and thoughts and deeds'. And finally, holding to 'truth in the darkest hour', the artist promises that from this time on, he will 'sing to the glory of the Lord'. Is this Van Morrison as the Dylanesque missionary man, just waiting to fall into the loving arms of Sir Cliff, or is it Van the lover of gospel music who'll sing any lyric if it gets him into the zone of rapture?

The light jazz-pop of 'Did Ye Get Healed?' doesn't really provide an answer. Its lyrics — particularly the lines 'Sometimes, when the spirit moves me / I can do many wondrous things' — wouldn't seem out of place in a revivalist church meeting. At a less exalted level, its promotion of music therapy grew from the artist's association with the Wrekin Trust (the album was released around the same time as the Loughborough University conference). The question in the song's title, expressed less archaically, would mark the end of many a subsequent live concert — or sometimes the beginning, as on *A Night in San Francisco* — but the track itself neatly sums up the notion of music as a healing force that runs through Morrison's mid-career albums.

Both the jaunty mood of 'Did Ye Get Healed?' and its uplifting lyrics, the presence of the spirit making each day an improvement on the last, might have come, like the lyrics of 'The Mystery', straightout of the Kingdom Hall. When Van gets that feeling deep down in his soul, he's just got to get out there on the dance floor and show off his moves. His heart is not thinking and his head is not feeling. He wants to tell you how to contemplate the mystery, pray, and then get up in rapture and boogie all night long with the true believers.

IRISH HEARTBEAT
(June 1988)

▪ *Star of the County Down* ▪ *Irish Heartbeat* ▪ *Tá Mo Chleamhnas Déanta* ▪ *Raglan Road* ▪ *She Moved Through the Fair* ▪ *I'll Tell Me Ma* ▪ *Carrickfergus* ▪ *Celtic Ray* ▪ *My Lagan Love* ▪ *Marie's Wedding*

Around the time of *No Guru, No Method, No Teacher*, Van Morrison began experimenting with the production of vocal sounds during deep meditation, speaking in tongues and releasing sound without the intervention of thought or application of choice. What emerged from these investigations into the voice-that-lay-beyond-words was a kind of folk music. In response, from around 1986–87 he began to listen

A working man in his prime

with renewed interest to the traditional music of Scotland and Ireland.

It isn't surprising that such traditional sounds emerged from the core of the singer's being. While much has been made of his childhood exposure to black American popular music, the fact is that folk music had also been one of the dominant influences on Morrison's early life. His mother Violet, whose musical interests were no less passionate than those of George Morrison, her record-collecting husband, possessed a great love of folk music, and two generations on, her grand-daughter Shana would recall Violet singing 'Star of the County Down', 'Danny Boy' and 'I'll Tell Me Ma' to her as a child. And from his father's side, the young Van inherited a love of folk ballads, particularly those sung by the popular Irish tenor John McCormack.

Traditional Irish songs, which is what almost all the tracks on *Irish Heartbeat* are, are built on two often interrelated themes: expatriation and repatriation, and the torment of love lost and found. These were, of course, themes that Morrison himself had explored throughout his career, and given that his work in the 1980s represented a slow-burning search for home, it was perhaps inevitable that he would consummate his return by making an album of Irish folk music.

The musical seeds of the *Irish Heartbeat* project were there from the moment that the tin whistle entered *Veedon Fleece* fourteen years before. *Into the Music*'s 'Rolling Hills' pointed the way forward, and progressively the songs from the early 1980s, with their Irish lyrics and occasional uillean pipes, made it clear that folk music was where some essential

Cry for home (1975–1991)

part of Van Morrison's musical personality lay. (This reached an early climax in the tracks recorded with Moving Hearts for *A Sense of Wonder*.)

By the time Van came to record with them, the Chieftains were an Irish institution and their role on the album, inevitably, was much more than that of a 'backing band'. Their first album had been recorded as early as 1964, although they only became a full-time act in 1975, the same year they achieved international prominence through their work on the Oscar-winning soundtrack to Stanley Kubrick's *Barry Lyndon*. In 1979 they played before 1.3 million people at an outdoor mass in Dublin, as 'support act' for Pope John Paul II, and in the year after *Irish Heartbeat*, they were made official national musical ambassadors by the Irish government. Built around original members Paddy Moloney (uillean pipes, tin whistle), Martin Fay (fiddle, percussion), and multi-instrumentalist Derek Bell (harp, percussion, keyboards, dulcimer, oboe), they would subsequently make a speciality out of collaborations with celebrities from outside the folk tradition.

Morrison had a fleeting encounter with the Chieftains as early as 1980, in Edinburgh, and his friendship with Derek Bell meant that contact was maintained. Long before the actual *Irish Heartbeat* television special, and the concerts and recording dates of 1987 and 1988, Morrison and the Chieftains' leader Paddy Moloney had already discussed making a joint album (as the band was to do in 1986 with classical flautist James Galway, and thereafter with countless other pop musicians). But initially nothing came of it. Then a handful of songs put together by a green-shirted Van and an inspired band of Chieftains went to air on St Patrick's Day

A working man in his prime

1987, and the project was clearly a goer. The *Irish Heartbeat* collaboration was to prove an inspiration to all concerned, and the resulting album and tour achieved perhaps more universal acclaim (except, surprisingly, in the United States) than anything that either party had done previously.

For many, Morrison singing the folk music of his native land unravelled a mystery. This was the essential voice and this was the thematic world that had lurked in the background, almost like a kind of template, through countless lyrics and tunes of love and spiritual searching. More than that, the project also allowed Morrison to share the stage with fellow legends — something that, as time would prove, often brought out the best in him. In that first television special, he was able to hide behind the drum kit, happily singing and playing away like Levon Helm — just another member of the band rather than a world-famous solo performer. Soon, he would almost always have a 'foil' like this, with first Georgie Fame, then Brian Kennedy and other guest artists, not to mention shades and dark hat to disguise Van the star as Van the working musician plying his trade among others. The Chieftains experience, while never repeated in the studio except for the occasional guest appearance on each other's album tracks, formed the climax of Morrison's period of homecoming, and opened up possibilities and techniques for future survival in the business that he loathed.

Pointedly, there were no new songs written for the album — it's about the past rather than the future — and the Morrison originals chosen for inclusion are two of his most explicit songs about returning home, drawn from *Beautiful Vision* and *Inarticulate Speech of the Heart*. The album's title track is all about going back to spend time 'with your own ones', while 'Celtic Ray' calls out to all the expatriate children of the British Isles to return home too. The static, haunting version of 'She Moved Through the Fair' probes typical John McCormack territory, while Violet Morrison's favourites are plundered for the spirited 'Star of the County Down' and the jaunty single, 'I'll Tell Me Ma'. 'Tá Mo Chleamhnas Déanta', a Gaelic tune, and the Scottish song, 'Marie's Wedding', also show off the chemistry between soloist and ensemble.

But really the album is built around the theme of love gone wrong, with Morrison's readings of 'Carrickfergus', 'My Lagan Love' and especially Patrick Kavanagh's 'Raglan Road', in which a hapless lover discovers too late that he has wooed 'a creature made of clay'. Not that the interpretations are without curiosity. In typical Van Morrison fashion, phrases are repeated over and over, and sometimes it sounds more like Ray Charles singing than an Irishman. But whenever Van seems likely to go over the top (as in 'My reason, my reason, my reason must allow'), the band chimes in and the Irish element is cranked up a notch.

There is something uplifting, not just about the music itself, but about the fact that this popular success was the most tangible musical outcome of that long journey homeward that had started twenty years earlier. Even better that Van Morrison, the professional performer and curmudgeon, seemed happier on stage than he'd ever been. Within the narrow confines of *Irish Heartbeat*'s folk sensibility, he appeared as a complete artist, comfortable with the material, individual in voice, and having a good time in the music of his 'own ones'.

A working man in his prime

AVALON SUNSET
(June 1989)

- Whenever God Shines His Light ▪ Contacting My Angel
- I'd Love to Write Another Song ▪ Have I Told You Lately
- Coney Island ▪ I'm Tired, Joey Boy ▪ When Will I Ever Learn to Live in God? ▪ Orangefield ▪ Daring Night
- These are the Days

Van Morrison's albums of the 1980s were notable for their consistency. Even the mixed-bags like *Inarticulate Speech of the Heart* and *A Sense of Wonder* contained some fine songs and moreover represented important landmarks or transition points along an important artistic path, which culminated in the sequence of three albums from *No Guru, No Method, No Teacher* through *Poetic Champions Compose* and on to *Irish Heartbeat*. No one could be expected to keep up the standard on an annual basis, however.

Virtually every song on *Avalon Sunset* replays ideas foreshadowed in the last three albums, if not earlier. While this extensive self-quotation inevitably suggests creative burnout, the results were convincing on a commercial level. The saccharine ballad 'Have I Told You Lately', for instance, will last for as long as easy-listening radio (and Rod Stewart) finds an audience, and the trivial duet with Cliff Richard, 'Whenever God Shines His Light', remains one of the biggest UK hits of Morrison's career. Other tracks that induce a sense of deja vu include the autobiographical 'Orangefield' and the equally nostalgic 'Coney Island', which has since been plundered by commercial advertisers and brought tears to the

Cry for home (1975–1991)

eyes of expatriate Ulstermen everywhere. And all four tracks were deemed suitably radio-friendly for single release — an unprecedented number of singles off a Van Morrison album. No one should begrudge him this success, though. After all, the string of first-rate records, each advancing on the ideas contained in the last, had earned their creator a commercial pay-off. It's difficult to know whether Morrison saw it this way during the making of the album, now for the Polydor label, but certainly the appearance of Cliff and Georgie Fame (on Hammond organ) added some star clout to the musician credits. Also in attendance at the various sessions in Bath and London were backing singers Katie Kissoon and Carol Kenyon, Irish guitar legend Arty McGlynn, bassist Clive Culbertson and drummer Dave Early, the last of whom, like some of the new faces at the *Poetic Champions* sessions, was a regular Morrison sideman in this period through to the early '90s.

And so to the songs that make up his first album of all-original material since 1986. The simple born-again message of 'Whenever God Shines His Light', with its stuttering riff, demands little analysis. Reach out for Him and He'll be there. While the idea of Morrison's partnership with Cliff Richard might have seemed unlikely to some, the Irishman had been a long-time fan and Richard had invited him to attend his revivalist meetings for arts workers. Morrison was a good candidate, not just because of his inexhaustible religious curiosity, but also because at the time he was writing straight-out devotional numbers like 'The Mystery' and 'Give Me My Rapture'. The spirit and the explicitly Christian sentiment expressed in 'Whenever God Shines His Light' could have appeared comfortably alongside those tracks on *Poetic Champions Compose*.

The Van Morrison phrasebook that lay open for 'Contacting My Angel' provided an encounter with a 'radiant' presence and a 'youth of a thousand summers', linking the latter to the eternal youth motif of *No Guru*. Elsewhere, it appends an opaque reference to Tennessee Williams with the repeated phrase 'sweet bird of youth' which dwells 'in my soul in my soul in my soul'.

The jazzy 'I'd Love to Write Another Song' is another of those writer's-block numbers — a song about not being able to write a song — the most distinguished predecessor of which was 'Tore Down à la Rimbaud' from *A Sense of Wonder*. But of course Morrison can and does write another song, seven more on this album in fact.

'Have I Told You Lately' includes some rather obvious rhymes ('love you'/'above you'), a promise, on behalf of the singer and his lover, to 'pray to the One', and a simple, hymn-like melody, reminiscent in style of 'Tupelo Honey'. At the time, it was probably the most mainstream ballad that Morrison had ever written. You could imagine Val Doonican singing it. You could almost imagine John McCormack singing it. Initially it was hard to imagine Rod Stewart singing it, but in hindsight no one should be surprised at anything he does by way of wasting one of the greatest rock 'n' roll voices in history. The song itself, like most of the others on *Avalon Sunset*, suggests that Morrison was rapidly squandering his own talents.

'Coney Island' is another one of those interminable Celtic-sounding instrumentals, but with a nostalgic poem about a childhood journey recited over the top. With its checklist of

Northern Ireland locations (Downpatrick, Strangford Lough, Shrigley, Killyleagh, the Lecale district, Ardglass and, of course, Coney Island itself) and foodstuffs (mussels, potted herrings), it's another Morrison litany set amid the predictable 'autumn sunshine'. It ends with the wish that the world should always be as it was during this perfect day's outing, 'And It Stoned Me' for the New Age.

In this context, 'I'm Tired, Joey Boy' might be thought to summarise the album as a whole. Sung to a shepherd (and given their traditional association with innocence and the pure, simple life, it's surprising that there aren't more shepherds in Morrison's songs), this is a complaint about life being 'so troubled' that it can only be assuaged by work. Specifically, it's the 'makings of men' that cause the problems, and the old misanthrope can only dream of being 'cheerful again'. On the one hand, his ambition takes him 'too far'; on the other, conservatism bores him. His solution — as always — is to go down to the river to 'watch the stream flow' and, more revealingly, to 'recall all the dreams that you once used to know'.

Once, of course, Van Morrison went to the river to dream. Now, in creative fatigue, he goes there to *re-create* the dreams he used to have. Middle age has hit, and he looks back on his past life and the pastures that weren't greener but meaner (presumably both America and the record industry.) At the conclusion of 'I'm Tired, Joey Boy', the resolution comes in cliché: he'll go up to the mountain once more (or alternatively the glen), where the silence can be found and the healing will begin (specifically, 'heartbreak will mend'). Somehow it's all just a bit pat now. The journey and the quest have become routine, the landmarks along the way too

A working man in his prime

familiar, and the path leads straight down the middle of the road.

But just when it seems that Morrison's greatcoat has been replaced by slippers and pipe, the music picks up in the second half of the album. 'When Will I Ever Learn to Live in God?' marks a return to the frustrated religious quest that dominated *No Guru*, and with its refreshing absence of spiritual certainty it brings some much-needed new imagery. At the outset, the sun is setting over Avalon — not the Irish landscape that we've encountered in the previous albums, but a return to England and the Arthurian landscape of *Common One*. Sitting in the West Country ('the last time we stood in the west'), Avalon was not just Morrison's geographic home at the time but also the place where Joseph of Arimathea supposedly commenced his English ministry. Its history and its mythology date back a millennium or more, functioning in Morrison's mind as the quintessential haunt of ancient peace.

The garbled third and fourth lines of the first verse, though, are revealing. 'Suffering long time angels enraptured by Blake / Burn out the dross innocence captured again' conflates several longstanding preoccupations: Blake's mystical vision of innocence, merged with Morrison's own fascination with sexual and heavenly angels, and Alice Bailey's theosophical notion of burning ground. Blake, Bailey and lovers in the English countryside — the recurrent inspirations during the period from *Common One* through to *No Guru*, and he wants them back. There is even a return to the harbour imagery of 'Almost Independence Day'.

But then, it's brought to his attention that everything (specifically art and architecture) is 'made in God' and this truth is eternal, but you have to gain access to it in 'your own way'. Morrison's 'own way' is to head back up that mountain-side again, where the shepherds are, where it's green and — as we well remember — where there's 'a sense of wonder'. A song that had started out quite promisingly ends in all the usual motifs.

Like so much else on this going-through-the-motions album, on a purely musical level 'Orangefield' sounds fine, with an engaging melody and curious sense of drama. But the lyrics are riddled with Morrison clichés. There's a 'golden autumn day' in the first line, and before the first verse is finished, the lover is spied 'standing by the riverside'. After the predictable set-up, nothing much happens. It's a simple love song to 'the apple of my eye', and she's in Orangefield, the scene of his childhood education.

The one track on the album that explores something like new territory is 'Daring Night'. Generating a real sense of momentum, the song takes the dancing-in-the-moonlight imagery common to several of Morrison's earlier songs and inflates it alarmingly. This is no moondance; this time we are out among the stars. The repeated reference to 'the Lord of the Dance' makes use of the title of Sydney Carter's famous song in order to draw on a medieval image of some complexity. Jesus Christ is the Lord of the Dance, the dancing in question standing for his life on earth. In the medieval lyric 'Tomorrow Shall Be My Dancing Day', Jesus invites his 'true love' (humankind) to join him in 'the general dance'. Morrison's version of this dance has a particular urgency about it — 'Don't let go', he repeatedly warns — and it is frankly cosmic in nature, a 'galactic swirl in the firmament'. The propulsive quality of the music is enhanced by Morrison's unusual vocal: he doesn't so much sing this song as *roar* it. It is a powerful noise, and the words are almost totally indistinct. Diction was never Morrison's strongest suit, but on 'Daring Night' he sounds as though he's recovering from extensive dental work, the muscles of his mouth numb and unresponsive. In addition, the voice is placed so far back in the mix that it is in permanent danger of being drowned out. So the overall impression is of the singer at the centre of this 'galactic swirl', roaring his exhilaration, but never in control.

Nothing among the earlier tracks on *Avalon Sunset* has prepared the listener for 'Daring Night', and the album's final song brings only bathos. After a collection that dredges up little but memories and images from the past, Morrison has the temerity to proclaim: 'There is no past, there's only future'. And then he runs through much of the catalogue of stock phrases one more time. 'These are the Days' begins with 'endless summer' and moves on to 'radiant heart', 'song of glory', 'sparkling river' and praise for 'the one great magician' who 'turned water into wine'.

Those listeners that had only heard and enjoyed *Irish Heartbeat* were no doubt thrilled by *Avalon Sunset*'s package of Irish mysticism and pop hits, just as they would be with the subsequent greatest-hits collection that took care to avoid Morrison's more extreme music (although it did include a rarity in the Robbie Robertson–produced 'Wonderful Remark', from the soundtrack of Martin Scorsese's *The King of Comedy*). Meanwhile, those with a more extensive knowledge of Van the Man's career could only smile patiently, enjoy the classic 'Daring Night', and wait for next year's offering.

Cry for home (1975–1991)

It is said that Charlie Chaplin once entered a Charlie Chaplin lookalike competition and came third. On *Avalon Sunset*, Van Morrison gave a credible impersonation of himself, but missed the main prize because others had learned how to 'be' Van too. The first single, 'Whenever God Shines His Light', received more radio attention than Morrison was used to, but the album's greatest success was in Rod Stewart's later version of 'Have I Told You Lately', which became a huge hit. With new fans still arriving through doors opened by collaborators Cliff Richard and Georgie Fame, Morrison had become an industry, the artist himself presiding over a mass production of the very things that had once made him unique.

ENLIGHTENMENT
(October 1990)

■ *Real Real Gone* ■ *Enlightenment* ■ *So Quiet in Here* ■ *Avalon of the Heart* ■ *See Me Through* ■ *Youth of 1,000 Summers* ■ *In the Days Before Rock 'n' Roll* ■ *Start All Over Again* ■ *She's My Baby* ■ *Memories*

The advent of Georgie Fame as a regular and significant contributor to Van Morrison's recordings and live shows brought with it a certain stabilising influence, which at the creative level was both a blessing and a curse. Undoubtedly, Fame's presence as an alternative frontman — or at least a stage foil — freed Van Morrison, to some extent, from his star duties, and the performances from 1990 onwards were notable for their joy and the comparative social acceptability of the singer's behaviour. But with Fame and guitarist Ronnie Johnson providing such solid and measured support, the music itself became more formulaic. Change the cover art and the title tracks and there would be little difference between the 'sound' of *Avalon Sunset* and that of its successor. *Enlightenment* might have used a few more musicians and been recorded in a different mix of English studios, but both albums are filled with production-line numbers as the Morrison conveyor belt rolls on into the new decade.

'The first song, 'Real Real Gone', is a classic belter in the tradition of 'Domino' and 'Wild Night', the title track continues the mystical quest for enlightenment, 'So Quiet in Here' searches for silence, 'Avalon of the Heart' is another search for the Holy Grail, and so on, through another 'Youth of 1,000 Summers', and a homage to the days before rock 'n' roll. All of these songs incorporate familiar lyrics, name-checks and self-quotations. Unmistakeably commercial in orientation, *Enlightenment* is, at least in its first half, Morrison Lite, designed to give the paying public more of what it wants in an inoffensive and easily digestible form.

'Real Real Gone' is boisterous, fresh and exciting — no mean achievement considering that the song itself was over a decade old (having originally been intended for inclusion on *Common One*). The protagonist might be drunk or spiritually abandoned. Whichever, he 'can't stand up by [himself]', he needs help, having been 'hit by a bow and arrow'. Of course this could also be Cupid firing darts, in which case the friend Morrison calls upon is presumably his new lover. But none of these ideas is pursued in any detail because one of Morrison's heroes, Sam Cooke, is on the radio and the singer winds up preaching the ministry of soul with quasi-biblical quotations of famous lines from those prophets Wilson Pickett, Solomon Burke, James Brown and Gene Chandler.

Just as the soul Sunday school learning-by-rote fades out, we hear those familiar New Age Celtic harmonies, like a synthetic choir, for the start of 'Enlightenment'. While we drift off into the mystic, Van enters with his Zen handbook, contemplating chopping wood, carrying water and the sound of one hand clapping. Its purpose? To protest that he — popular music's most determined spiritual searcher — hasn't any idea what enlightenment is. Perhaps he was simply trying to put interpreters and critics off the scent. In any case, the spiritual doubt that had emerged in *No Guru, No Method, No Teacher* here becomes an ill-tempered rant about giving up because the thing he's been searching for 'keeps changing to something different'. With the spiritual goalposts moving, the formerly resolute searcher can only hope for 'non-attachment' to the Jehovah's Witnesses, Rosicrucians, Scientologists, Theosophists, Alice Bailey acolytes, Zen masters, Krishna devotees and even the sexual partners who had directed him on his various quests. The only solution is 'making your own reality', and ultimately religious or spiritual enlightenment is 'up to you' and 'the way you think'. On the philosophical level it's at best rather unenlightening and, at worst, a slap in the face for fellow searchers. From an aesthetic perspective, it's simply not resonant. 'It's up to you' explicitly dumps the listener as baggage in the song. But the tune is great.

More rewarding for those who know Van the Man's music well is 'So Quiet in Here', with a motoring rhythm track and lyrics that begin with the line 'Foghorns blowing in the night', an obvious throwback to the imagery of 'Into the Mystic' from twenty years before. The opening verse is confusing though, because we're in a car driving along the coastline, yet the refrain 'So quiet in here' suggests we're simultaneously indoors. Certainly there's a candle lighting up the lover's face in verse two, so it seems that the 'paradise' being described is actually an interior. After all the singer's 'struggling in the world' and 'so many dreams that don't come true', he's able to put the problems aside and simply enjoy the heavenly moment with his lover. Then we get an alternative perspective on paradise, which becomes a glass of wine with friends and 'talking into the wee hours of the dawn', before the song heads back to the ocean, with ships moving off into the night to a place 'where we can be what we wanna be'. It's been a while since Morrison had written about going away rather than coming home, but here in arguably the best — and certainly the most characteristic — song on the album, he sets sail again into the mystic. For a brief moment, we remember what it was like when he was doing it for real.

'Avalon of the Heart' quotes directly from the preceding album's title track so it's not easy to believe the song's message that 'the journey has only just begun' and that he's 'making a brand new start'. Against the backdrop of Fiachra Trench's lush string arrangement, the Holy Grail appears 'behind the sun' (if that's possible) and then we're right back to *Astral Weeks*, with the enchanted vale emerging 'down by the viaducts of my dreams'. This also happens to be 'down by Camelot', but the mental geography has now become confused and it's unclear whether the mythical world shaping the musical rapture is Arthurian or Lewis Merensteinian.

Cry for home (1975–1991)

Fortunately, the issue is resolved in the second half of 'Avalon of the Heart'. The cup from which Christ drank at the Last Supper (that is, 'in the upper room') and which was souvenired by Joseph of Arimathea now makes its appearance, according to legend in Avalon, there in the English West Country. Morrison is replaying the opening of Blake's 'Jerusalem', picking up on the question 'And did those feet in ancient times, walk upon England's mountains green?'. Christ himself might not have, but in Morrison's version, Joseph and the cup certainly did. Perhaps because he had a home of his own in Somerset, he appears to have swallowed the legend hook, line and sinker, and in the song it's so ingrained in his heart that it inspires him to make another of those brand new starts. But it isn't explained just what this start is. Certainly it's nothing new musically, because the songs that follow are a puzzling and half-hearted collection, and all of them look back to better times.

'See Me Through' is a reworking of 'Real Real Gone', even employing the very word 'gone' again (as in drunk as a skunk). The singer needs someone to lean on, and, supporting the 'drinking' interpretation of both songs, there are references to the Alcoholics Anonymous pledge of 'One day at a time', while the phrase 'days of wine and roses' might be a reference to the film featuring Jack Lemmon as a recovering alcoholic. A bit more self-quotation ensues, this time going right back to Them's 'Baby, Please Don't Go', before Van remembers himself as a schoolboy — 'before TV, before rock 'n' roll, previous, previous . . .'.

The fade-out of 'See Me Through' might have segued neatly into 'In the Days Before Rock 'n' Roll', but instead the days of eternal youth are resurrected in another song built exclusively out of Morrison clichés. The title itself, 'Youth of 1,000 Summers' was used as a lyric on the preceding album and its idea had permeated *No Guru*. From there, we go through the second use of Tennessee Williams's 'Sweet Bird of Youth' in as many albums, and another grab-bag of Morrison favourites, including 'in my soul' repeated over and over again, radiance and shining 'like the sun', mountains, a 'clear crystal fountain', rivers, and a reappearance of the Ancient of Days, skipping, dancing and singing. A comedian couldn't have constructed a better parody of a Van Morrison song: there is literally nothing else in the lyric but these clichés. Anyone looking for signs that Van the Man was burnt out would probably rest their case right here.

'In the Days Before Rock 'n' Roll' offers yet more nostalgia and the Irish poet (and co-writer) Paul Durcan's self-important vocal is possibly the most irritating thing ever recorded on a Van Morrison album. The song, which lasts an interminable fifteen minutes, is sometimes hailed as the definitive Morrison childhood epic, but this is surely only because it's a literal recollection of the pirate radio stations that inspired the singer in the 1950s. It's also the most extensive list of names, with Fats, Elvis, Sonny, Lightnin', Muddy, John Lee, Ray Charles, Jerry Lee Lewis and Little Richard all receiving brief but fawning acknowledgement. But for all those explicit references to soul and rock stars, while tuning into Radio Luxembourg and many other radio stations, the song nevertheless contains some classic Morrison obfuscations. Jockey Lester Piggott gets a mention, for instance, there's a mystifying line about letting the goldfish go (presumably releasing a wild creature back into a clear

Cry for home (1975–1991)

mountain stream), and the song itself is built around speculations about what one 'Justin' is up to now. Perhaps this Justin was a pirate radio DJ, but who would know? (Durcan himself once confessed that he didn't.) There's just too much self-indulgence for any listener to care. In short, 'In the Days Before Rock 'n' Roll' is a woeful travesty in which the twiddling of knobs isn't confined to the radio dial alone.

The album never really recovers. Whereas the first half could at least be described as a summation of the artist's predominant themes, the second offers only nonsense and clichés, the like of which hadn't been seen since *Tupelo Honey*. 'Start All Over Again' returns to 'Avalon of the Heart's' theme of renewal, but its big-band feel fails to compensate for a lack of conviction or useful meaning in the lyrics. For genuine verbal ineptitude, however, it can't compete with 'She's My Baby', with its rhymes of 'blue'/'thinking of you', 'high'/'sky', 'low'/'go' and plenty of similar banalities. Were Van Morrison not singing it, the song would surely have been trashed.

And then the album peters out with 'Memories', which is a timid replay of *Avalon Sunset*'s 'These are the Days', with Morrison proclaiming unnecessarily that memories are all that he has. With the lack of inspiration or new ideas so sadly demonstrated on *Enlightenment*, 'Memories' effectively summarises the artist's situation at that point in his career.

For all the strident claims that *Enlightenment* makes about a 'brand new start', everything about the album looks back to more inspired times. And as in *Avalon Sunset*, we're left wondering whether this great artist still has it in him to move forward, or whether the lucrative world of the nostalgia market now beckons all too enticingly.

A working man in his prime

HYMNS TO THE SILENCE
(September 1991)

▪ *Professional Jealousy* ▪ *I'm Not Feeling it Anymore* ▪ *Ordinary Life* ▪ *Some Peace of Mind* ▪ *So Complicated* ▪ *I Can't Stop Loving You* ▪ *Why Must I Always Explain?* ▪ *Village Idiot* ▪ *See Me Through Part II (Just a Closer Walk With Thee)* ▪ *Take Me Back* ▪ *By His Grace* ▪ *All Saints Day* ▪ *Hymns to the Silence* ▪ *On Hyndford Street* ▪ *Be Thou My Vision* ▪ *Carrying a Torch* ▪ *Green Mansions* ▪ *Pagan Streams* ▪ *Quality Street* ▪ *It Must Be You* ▪ *I Need Your Kind of Loving*

Given that *Enlightenment* had been an exercise in repetition, with half a side featuring Morrison running on empty, the decision within a year to release not just another collection but the first studio double album of his career looked to be a misjudgement. On recent efforts it seemed that there just wasn't enough creative spark to sustain a 45-minute collection of new material, let alone double that. And that's exactly how it proved on *Hymns to the Silence*.

Still, for the musicians who regularly backed the singer in the studio during this period, the continued prodigious output kept them in regular employment. Indeed, keyboard players Georgie Fame and Neil Drinkwater, bassist Steve Pearce, drummer Dave Early, saxophonist Steve Gregory, singers Katie Kissoon and Carol Kenyon, and arranger Fiachra Trench must all have been coming to appreciate that, once you were 'in' with Van the Man, it was close to a full-time gig. Joining this list at the sessions for Morrison's twentieth studio album (including the collaboration with the Chieftains) was bassist Nicky Scott, who would feature on many of the Ulsterman's projects through to *What's Wrong With This Picture?* in 2003.

Giving truth to the old adage that quantity is no guarantee of quality, almost half of *Hymns to the Silence* consists of whingeing songs that are uninspired at the lyrical level, and only one of which bears any sign of musical inspiration. Worse than that, the lyrics of these songs of complaint and self-pity reveal such a mean-spiritedness and contempt for the devoted fan that they appear not just lacking in dignity, style and class, but much worse, utterly devoid of the bite, word play and rapier wit that make the hate songs of Bob Dylan such impressive artistic achievements.

This predominance of oh-woe-is-me material is a pity because in certain places *Hymns to the Silence* provides a profound perspective on some of Morrison's perennial themes. The title track is no 'Listen to the Lion', but its musical appeal is similarly compelling and hypnotic, while 'On Hyndford Street' finds the childhood reminiscences reinvigorated and unusually articulate. And the album's two diversions into actual hymn tunes ('Be Thou My Vision' and 'Just a Closer Walk with Thee' as part of 'See Me Through Part II') represent a genuinely new direction with the potential to open up a whole new genre for the singer — a development that hasn't been explored further outside this sprawling effort.

But those moments of inspiration are a long way ahead as the album kicks off with a suite of complaints about the misery of being famous. In 'Professional Jealousy' we learn that 'personal invasion can ruin a man' and are reminded again of 'the price that he's paying' for doing what he does.

A working man in his prime

The diction embraces the mood of the song, with keywords including 'abuse', 'lie', 'sin', 'bitter', 'angry' and 'crazy'. It's strange that such heated language is cast in an innocuous r&b context, especially when one considers that at this time, rather more urgent songs of loathing were emerging from Kurt Cobain in Seattle, with thrilling brute force and primal energy.

'I'm Not Feeling it Anymore' covers the same territory, the gist being that 'If this is success then something's awful wrong'. Beginning with an acknowledgement of the need (as in *No Guru*) 'to get back to base', it concludes with the Beatles' observation that money can't buy you love, and also that 'the truth will set you free'. Everyone, whether a famous pop star or an only child, feels these things from time to time, but they remain difficult sentiments for an audience to embrace as its own. It just seems to be too much about the songwriter himself and not enough about the universal experience of grief and suffering.

The trouble with being Van Morrison finds a possible resolution in the pedestrian 'Ordinary Life', where a mundane existence is hailed as 'my rock in times of trouble'. The singer needs a woman who can lead this ordinary life with him and to help 'bring me down to earth' and 'keep my feet on the ground'. The ideas fuelling these kinds of thoughts are incontrovertible given the degree of fame that Morrison has achieved — why *wouldn't* he hanker after such normality? (Certainly, his return to being an ordinary, jobbing musician around this time, in the form of impromptu and anonymous gigs at the King's Hotel in Newport, south Wales, resulted in some of his most inspired live performances.) No doubt the frustration of stardom is justifiable. It's just that, when addressed directly and with such absence of subtlety or complexity, it doesn't make for an interesting song.

The complaints go on. In 'Some Peace of Mind', we learn how lonely it gets out on the road 'doing my job'; while in 'So Complicated' all he really wants to do is 'blow my horn'. He doesn't want to 'think about the business no more' but rather just get up and play. Good. Please do.

Don Gibson's 'I Can't Stop Loving You', a song made famous first by Ray Charles in 1962 and then Presley during his Vegas years, serves as another exercise in nostalgia, indirectly recalling the memories of 'happy hours so long ago' from *Irish Heartbeat*'s 'Carrickfergus'. When released as the album's first single in the UK, it carried the credit 'with the Chieftains', a reminder that it was the 1988 collaboration that relaunched the Ulsterman's career commercially in Britain.

The suite of misery then concludes with arguably its most offensive lyric but most interesting music in 'Why Must I Always Explain?', another song chosen as a single in Britain. Patrick Humphries and Clinton Heylin identify 'Tupelo Honey' as the source of the tune (they are harmonically similar but not melodically), and certainly the music shares its hymn-like quality. While Morrison's fans and business colleagues alike are being berated as 'hypocrites and parasites and people that drain', musically the song probes a fascinating blend of traditional styles. It's the Chieftains in church and with a less vitriolic lyric it could have been a major achievement.

Folk-music references continue in 'Village Idiot', an unlikely tale of an Irish idiot savant who, like Ol' Man River, 'must know something but he's just not saying'. The song develops the experience of working with the Chieftains, although, as in the previous song, those Irish legends of folk music don't actually appear. And if only because it's the first track that does not explicitly complain about the difficulty of being Van Morrison (at least, it's unlikely that the idiot in question is meant to be Morrison), it gains added force as the kind of song that would sound better in more tightly argued company — an album of Irish folk and hymn tunes, for instance.

At last the album is up and running, but the need for self-quotation again rears its ugly head in 'See Me Through Part II', wherein the lyrics from the *Enlightenment* song are reprised in the context of the hymn, 'Just a Closer Walk With Thee'. Despite the familiarity of the source material, here we find some innovation that could lead the artist forward, in the form of segues between numbers from vastly different styles. This device prepares the way for the inspired medley-fest of *A Night in San Francisco* a few years later, and it's an encouraging sign that Morrison hasn't lost his touch on this problematic double album after all. He's just taken a momentary pause to get a few gripes off his chest, whether or not anyone else wishes to hear them.

'Take Me Back' is another unintentional self-parody song (like those on *Avalon Sunset* and *Enlightenment*), in which all the favoured themes come and go in a guided tour of the 'Caledonian' genre: 'walking by the river', 'help me understand', 'Do you remember the time ... when everything made more sense in the world?', 'too much suffering and confusion', 'let me understand religion', 'you walked in a green field', 'down an avenue of trees', 'on a golden summer', 'the music on the radio', 'in the night-time while we're still and quiet', 'look out on the water and the big ships', 'we sat and listened to Sonny Boy blow', 'everything felt so good and right', 'when you lived in the light'. It moves towards meditation and resolves with 'In the light, in the grace / And the blessing', lyrics that, in a return to the technique used previously on *Veedon Fleece*, are then picked up on in the following track, which starts the second CD.

'By His Grace' is Van Morrison's first original devotional song. It takes the form of a spiritual handbook for those wishing to enter 'the kingdom on high', although, like 'See Me Through' on the previous album, it picks up on the AA line of 'One day at a time'. 'All Saints Day', which follows, isn't as religious as its title suggests, but just an engaging little number setting up an assignation on that day with a woman named Sue. It serves as an overture for the lengthy, distinctive and altogether marvellous meditative sequence that follows.

The title track is of little consequence lyrically, consisting of a minor love lyric involving absence and the repetition of key phrases. But the point of 'Hymns to the Silence' is to wind the album down into that characteristic space where meditation and contemplation can occur. Of course we go 'out in the countryside' and encounter the 'cool, clear crystal water' for the umpteenth time, but it doesn't matter because these phrases, and the mantra 'Close to the One' are intended only as a means to an end. We are headed for silence and memory, and while the song may not be the strongest Morrison meditation, it's evocative and hypnotic enough to usher in the major act of recovered memory that follows.

The glorious 'On Hyndford Street' is a straight autobiographical narration over typically hushed and dreamy

A working man in his prime

Celtic accompaniment (courtesy of Chieftain Derek Bell's synthesizer), but in it, Morrison writes arguably his most moving evocation of childhood, replete with multiple references to Belfast place names. As guru Van leads us back into that spellbinding world, we actually 'feel' the silence at half-past-eleven in the evening in that 1950s city where business and public transport all shut down early and people left the streets. The radio's playing and as voices drift over Beechie River, young Van is lying there 'dreaming, in God'. From there the memory indulges in free association, with scenes from the writer's childhood wafting over with occasionally curious allusions (did Van really listen to 'Debussy on the [BBC radio] Third Programme'?).

The reverie wouldn't be complete, of course, without some name-checks, and here 'Mr Jelly Roll', Big Bill Broonzy and Mezz Mezzrow join the more familiar Jack Kerouac, who makes his first appearance since 'Cleaning Windows' nine years before. Morrison's vocal delivery is so rapt, the memories so compelling, and the lead-up via the preceding songs so perfect that for once the clichés and repetition seem irrelevant. He has covered this territory plenty of times in the past, but here in this sublime song he gets it right.

The way out from the perfect musical moment is also inspirational, with a rendition of the old Protestant hymn 'Be Thou My Vision' stout and unemotional, and accompanied by another interjection of pipes and folk instruments courtesy of the Chieftains.

'Carrying a Torch' possesses an anthemic quality that's not so far removed from the hymn aesthetic that has sustained the non-complaint part of the album. Written for Tom Jones

Cry for home (1975–1991)

(and released as the title track of his 1991 album, which included three other songs from *Hymns*), the first verse of 'Carrying a Torch' veers dangerously close to another spilling of the guts about 'how much it costs' to keep carrying this damned torch. Fortunately, it heads in another direction before it's too late, with a celebration of the brightness with which the flame of love burns.

'Green Mansions' returns to familiar motifs. The image of a 'mansion on the hill' had been around since 'Cyprus Avenue' on *Astral Weeks*, even if, by this stage, it was more closely associated with Bruce Springsteen than with its originator. Alice Bailey is also back again, smiling beneficently over the song's quasi-mystical location, which is 'free from the glamour of the world'. But at least, after all that initial complaining, *Hymns to the Silence* has finally lifted its gaze, via meditation, to burning torches held aloft and mansions in lofty places 'where the story does unfurl'.

'Pagan Streams' then retraces the steps of the meditative section of the album, and the clichés are rolled out yet again. There's the white horse that graced the cover of *Tupelo Honey* (hence, perhaps, the song's refrain 'on Honey Street'?), and once all noise abates, we get back in touch with silence, meditation and contemplation as we stand on a hillside with — you guessed it — 'a sense of wonder'. And in this familiar landscape, Morrison develops his 'Ordinary Life' scenario by dreaming of becoming a bee-keeper (just as Bob Dylan had lamented that if only he'd been a doctor, he might have 'done some good in the world'). Here in this career-change fantasy, perhaps we might locate the origin of the old line 'Just like honey baby . . .'.

But then we're back to the formula. Dr John's 'Quality Street' bounces along in standard territory ('I thank God for sending me you'), while 'It Must Be You' is filled with mundane sentiments elaborated vocally by repeated 'baby baby baby's and 'really do believe's.

The third and last of these back-to-back nondescript love songs is the album closer, 'I Need Your Kind of Loving'. Here, the fortunes of love are paralleled with meteorological changes ('Well, my baby's gone, so's summer', 'Well, I love you in the springtime / When the rippling streams begin to flow') until, in a nod to Chuck Berry's telecommunications heartbreak of 'Memphis Tennessee', he begs: 'Operator, operator / Put me through to my baby now'. In all, it's an innocuous ending to an album.

Perhaps more than any of his other works, *Hymns to the Silence* demonstrates the good, the bad and the ugly sides of Van Morrison. Some years earlier he had come home, and while the struggle to get there had inspired much of his finest work, his arrival was the worst thing that could have happened. Once at home, the only thing left for Morrison to do was reflect on the adventure from the comfort of an armchair, with the devoted attention of loyal listeners still willing to hear it all over again.

ON WITH THE SHOW
(1992–2003)

■ *Too Long in Exile* ■ *Days Like This* ■ *The Healing Game* ■
Back on Top ■ *Down the Road* ■ *What's Wrong With This
Picture?*

The eleven studio albums that Morrison released beginning with *Into the Music* in 1979 and ending with *Hymns to the Silence* twelve years later shared the common theme of homecoming, more or less strongly present from record to record. For more than a decade, Van Morrison came home to Ireland. The promise of 'Almost Independence Day' was kept again and again. The next album represented a different sort of homecoming, however. This was Van reuniting not so much with Ireland as with his musical youth, with the blues, with jazz, with John Lee Hooker, even with his first big hit, 'Gloria'.

    The new record ushered in a period in which Morrison would re-examine his musical roots in detail, with albums that were bluesier or jazzier than anything in his back catalogue

A working man in his prime

and tribute albums to Mose Allison, the country blues (through the skiffle of Lonnie Donegan) and country and western songs. In passing, he appeared as a guest on albums by several more of his heroes, including the Holmes Brothers, John Lee Hooker, the Chieftains, B. B. King, Carl Perkins and Ray Charles. This period would culminate in Morrison being signed to the jazz label, Blue Note, bringing his career full-circle with an album of pure show-band repertoire, entitled *What's Wrong with This Picture?* (2003).

The answer to a question posed by that particular album, as much as anything, was that, as he approached the age of 60, Morrison seemed to have abandoned his spiritual searching. After *The Healing Game* (1997), one of his finest and most underrated records, he suddenly appeared to have the answers.

TOO LONG IN EXILE
(June 1993)

- *Too Long in Exile* ▪ *Big Time Operators* ▪ *Lonely Avenue* ▪ *Ball & Chain* ▪ *In the Forest* ▪ *Till We Get the Healing Done* ▪ *Gloria* ▪ *Good Morning Little Schoolgirl* ▪ *Wasted Years* ▪ *The Lonesome Road* ▪ *Moody's Mood for Love* ▪ *Close Enough for Jazz [instrumental]* ▪ *Before the World Was Made* ▪ *I'll Take Care of You* ▪ *Instrumental* ▪ *Tell Me What You Want*

It had been almost two years since *Hymns to the Silence* and, for an album-a-year man such as Van Morrison, that must have seemed 'too long not singing my song', to quote from the title track of this 1993 release. Specifically the song that Van had not been singing, following a decade or more exploring his Celtic roots, was the blues. *Hymns* had had its share of r&b, but not on the scale of *Too Long in Exile*, which seemed on release to contain the bluesiest side of Morrison since *It's Too Late to Stop Now*, the live album of 1974.

In keeping with this new approach to album content, the making of *Too Long in Exile* saw some major changes in the production process. Although much of this collection was recorded, as usual, at Bath's Wool Hall Studios, for the first time since 1986's *No Guru, No Method, No Teacher*, sessions were also held outside England or Ireland, back at Sausalito. And while Georgie Fame, Nicky Scott and Kate St John were retained from his most recent projects, many of the musicians that had regularly backed the singer since *Poetic Champions Compose* were now gone.

Beginning an album with its title track for the first time since *Astral Weeks* was a gesture not lost on Van Morrison's fans, many of whom rushed to speak of *Too Long in Exile* as a return to form. (Every subsequent album of original material has been greeted in the same way, titles such as *The Healing Game* and *Back on Top* only adding to the impression that an artistic renaissance is under way.) And sure enough, after a stuttering drum roll, there is Van telling us that he's been away too long, while the band and backing vocalists, a spring in their step, saunter though a sort of good-humoured shuffle. But 'Too Long in Exile' doesn't really deliver. At six minutes, its slim musical content is over-extended and we end up being subjected to one of Morrison's more predictable lists, this time of other Irishmen — major literary figures and temperamental sporting heroes — who were themselves 'too long in exile'.

After the unsatisfying first track, the next begins promisingly, a twelve-bar blues. Morrison half sings, half talks his way through 'Big Time Operators', enumerating the injustices perpetrated by them (presumably the Bernses) on a 'young and green' artist (presumably Van Morrison). If you didn't know the stories of Morrison's time in New York City in 1967, you might conclude that 'Big Time Operators' was the result of heavy-duty paranoia, but most of the incidents described in the song do seem to have happened. The only paranoid aspect of the song is that a quarter of a century later, Morrison is still obsessed by it all.

Next up is 'Lonely Avenue', another twelve-bar blues. Written by Doc Pomus — of 'Youngblood', 'Save the Last Dance for Me' and 'Little Sister' fame — it was an r&b hit for Ray Charles in 1956. Almost forty years later, Morrison delivers a lazy smoulder of a performance.

From its title, 'Ball & Chain' sounds as if it should be yet another twelve-bar; it isn't though. It's a bright little pop tune in C major, but with words that make it one of the strangest love songs written by Morrison or anyone else. Although musically far removed from the blues, in its line structure it closely resembles the Willie Dixon song that was featured, memorably, on *It's Too Late to Stop Now*. In 'I Just Want to Make Love to You', the singer lists those things he doesn't want his lover to be (his slave, sad and blue) or do (make his bed, bake his bread), explaining that all he wants is to make love to her. In 'Ball & Chain', Morrison, like Dixon, begins line after line with the words 'I don't want', in the process making a list of all the things that don't interest him about the woman he is addressing. It's not that he finds her attractive, he says, or that he feels obliged to her or that she is rich or even that he loves her. No, in a return to the theme of 'Ordinary Life' from *Hymns to the Silence*, he wants her to be his ball and chain, someone to tie him down and restrict his freedom. He has, he tells us, been trying 'to find [his] way back home' but failed, again and again. He is destined to live out 'a fugitive dream', but this will end because he will see his lover 'in the garden once again', where she'll be 'standing in the summer rain'. In other words, despite the happy-go-lucky sound of the music, despite the blues references, and despite the apparently masochistic desire to be fitted out with a ball and chain, we are slipping back once more into classic Morrison mysticism.

It grows stronger, for 'Ball & Chain' is the first in a strange triptych of songs. Chained to his woman, the singer now finds himself in a new setting on 'In the Forest', which it soon transpires is rather like being 'in the garden'. Kate St John's cor anglais is even there, just as her oboe was in 1986. The forest, like the garden, is wet with 'summer rain', and Morrison intends to meet a woman there. She will be wearing 'long robes' and he will hold in his arms. Note that the song is set sometime in the future. The long robes suggest some ritual, but it is not clear what ritual that might be. Perhaps they're going to be married. Perhaps she is the 'ball and chain' of the previous track. At any rate, the two of them will 'surely roam' down by 'the ancient roads', and he promises to take her 'home to the forest'. At the end of the song, the cor anglais is joined by Candy Dulfer's saxophone and Morrison's wordless 'na na'-ing.

Which brings us to the third song in the sequence and to the heart of this curious album. 'Till We Get the Healing Done' takes over precisely where 'In the Forest' left off. Where previously they were making plans to 'roam down by the ancient roads', now they're heading 'down those ancient streets' and 'ancient roads', as a result of which, 'together' they will 'get the healing done'. Musically, this track couldn't be simpler. It consists of fifteen straight verses plus a coda. There is no middle eight, no variation to the harmony, just the sound of Morrison's voice building as the song continues on its long course. The first half of each verse is in E minor and has a descending motif; the second half is in the relative major of G, with a hopeful rising figure accompanying the repeated refrain of 'Till we get the healing done'.

The song is part litany, part mantra and part spiritual step plan, aiming at a series of enlightened states of mind and wellbeing. Along the way these include dwelling 'in the house of the Lord', living 'in the Light' and (proving that Morrison still recalls one of the central tenets from 'Christmas Humphrey's book on Zen') knowing 'your original face'. 'Till We Get the Healing Done' is also about keeping on and not giving up, and this is evident as much from the music as from the words. Indeed, notwithstanding the ecumenical religious references, Morrison's soulful performance becomes increasingly sexual in tone as it builds to a climax and, in the gentle fading coda, we hear that getting 'the healing done' will also involve his 'baby' staying 'all night long', even 'to the break of day'. If the connection with *Into the Music*'s 'And the Healing Has Begun' wasn't evident before, it is made manifest in this coda. Healing

On with the show (1992–2003)

might begin with Jesus and the Buddha, but a little backstreet jellyroll seals the deal.

So the 'ball and chain' wooed and wed, and the healing done, the party can commence. Although only the sixth song on an album of fifteen tracks, 'Till We Get the Healing Done's length of eight-and-a-half minutes means that we've now reached the halfway point. There's still forty minutes of this CD remaining, and it is, after all, meant to be a blues album. What better, then, than to strike up the opening chords of 'Gloria' and invite John Lee Hooker to sing it? This version of Morrison's classic is subtler than it was when Them recorded it nearly thirty years earlier, Hooker bringing a sort of querulous vulnerability to his performance, before Van joins in with some encouraging noises of his own. But who needs a subtle, querulous, vulnerable version of 'Gloria'? The general public, it seemed, judging by the decision to release this 1993 revamp as the album's only single.

'Good Morning Little Schoolgirl' follows, the track sequencing here implying that we've settled in for a true blues fest in the mid and late portion of the album. However, as with the preceding 'Gloria', the result is competent but uninspiring. Van would make soon amends on *A Night in San Francisco*, with a performance of this Sonny Boy Williamson classic that's so ardent, it makes you wonder if you should be phoning the cops.

Hooker returns for the next offering, 'Wasted Years'. Although it's listed as a Morrison original, this is just an anonymous-sounding, common-or-garden blues. True to the song's title, Van and John Lee trade phrases about suffering for four rather pointless minutes.

A working man in his prime

Aside from the fact that we've already had a similarly titled song earlier on in 'Lonely Avenue', the next track, Shilkret and Austin's 'The Lonesome Road', is a real oddity in the midst of all the blues and jazz that dominates the second half of *Too Long in Exile*. Nathaniel Shilkret was a composer and conductor in the Hollywood tradition, straddling film and classical music. (Shilkret, it was, who commissioned Arnold Schoenberg's *Prelude to the Genesis*.) 'The Lonesome Road' is not one of his most ambitious works, but a World War II pop song, in which Gene Austin's lyrics advise looking down 'that lonesome road' before opting to travel along it. It is an all-purpose show-band song, the versatility of which is amply demonstrated by the fact that, long before Morrison gave it his best shot, it had been sung by artists ranging from Paul Robeson and Frank Sinatra to Esther and Abi Ofarim.

Failing to heed that song's advice about looking before you leap, this album (already too long) now plunges headlong through a mini-suite of jazz tunes, beginning with saxophonist James Moody's famous gloss on the standard 'I'm in the Mood for Love'. Nothing impresses, and Morrison's misguided, if optimistic, stab at the tricky vocal line of 'Moody's Mood for Love' is particularly dismal. He hangs on valiantly, but pays scant regard to such technicalities as correct intonation, and sounds as though he is having a horrible time.

This fiasco is hardly helped by the anodyne instrumental that immediately follows, entitled, in an unwitting irony, 'Close Enough for Jazz'. Close but no cigar, and the party stalls again.

Next up, Morrison has a favourite poem by W.B. Yeats that he wants to share with us. He can't remember the words

On with the show (1992–2003)

exactly, but he has a go, singing 'Before the World Was Made' to a tune by Kenny Craddock (who was a keyboard player with Van's band briefly in the '80s). The most interesting thing about this song is the way that the singer extends Yeats's use of the Buddhist imagery. Yeats had written: 'I'm looking for the face I had / Before the world was made', to which Morrison adds, for the second time on this album, the phrase 'Your original face'.

And then it's into almost a quarter of an hour of more blues, with an undistinguished cover of Brook Benton's 'I'll Take Care of You' morphing into an untitled instrumental, which in turn moves on to 'Tell Me What You Want'. The last track — perhaps in an effort to reward the listener's patience — offers the come-ons 'Tell me what you want . . . tell me what you need'.

On the plus side, *Too Long in Exile* returned Van Morrison to the Top 30 of the US albums chart for the first time since 1978. But, as an ardent blues fan since childhood, and one of the few white exponents of the genre who can convince when performing alongside a genuine master, Morrison surely knew he'd failed to hit the mark. It cannot be a coincidence that within six months of this album's release, he took many of the same musicians — guitarist Ronnie Johnson, bassist Nicky Scott, drummer Geoff Dunn, organist John Savannah, multi-instrumentalist Teena Lyle and saxophonist Candy Dulfer — and recorded the second double live set of his career. Nor that among copious jazz and blues covers, *A Night in San Francisco* should contain fine accounts of three of the songs dealt with so half-heartedly here ('I'll Take Care of You', 'Good Morning Little Schoolgirl' and 'Lonely Avenue').

A working man in his prime

In the first of these, a tune once associated with Bobby 'Blue' Bland, Van takes off on one of his extended codas. 'I'm drifting, I'm drifting', he sings, until finally he drifts all the way into James Brown's 'It's a Man's, Man's, Man's World', where, as if to disprove the statement in the title, Ms Dulfer's sax solo burns brightly. Then it's straight into 'Lonely Avenue', except that there's nothing straight about this performance. Haji Ahkba's flugelhorn works itself into a small frenzy, Dulfer's alto builds on this and before you know it, Morrison and the band are passing through a range of only vaguely related material, some of it by Van himself, most of it not, before arriving back at 'Lonely Avenue'. Powerful stuff, then, and if *Too Long in Exile* had contained performances as good as these, it would count as a major work.

Too Long in Exile is an album one tends to misremember. Because so much of it is blues-orientated, and so much of that is frankly uninspiring, one thinks of the disc as a failed attempt to return to the music of Morrison's youth. Here is Van, in mid-life, trying to capture the spirit of those Ray Charles and Bobby 'Blue' Bland songs he used to perform with the Monarchs. Here is Van reviving 'Gloria', his biggest hit with Them. Here is Van, indeed, searching for his 'original face' in music. And, not to mince words, the results are boring. What is more, they distract our attention from the interesting three-song sequence at the heart of the album. 'Ball & Chain', 'In the Forest' and 'Till We Get the Healing Done' contain little that is musically exceptional, but there are few places in Morrison's work where the lyrics articulate so clearly the connections between home and healing, spirituality and sex.

On with the show (1992–2003)

DAYS LIKE THIS
(June 1995)

- Perfect Fit ▪ Russian Roulette ▪ Raincheck ▪ You Don't Know Me ▪ No Religion ▪ Underlying Depression ▪ Songwriter ▪ Days Like This ▪ I'll Never Be Free ▪ Melancholia ▪ Ancient Highway ▪ In the Afternoon

With *Too Long in Exile*, Van Morrison began a series of studio albums characterised by a close engagement with the blues and with jazz, by tributes to other musicians working in those areas, and by cover versions of much of their material. But *Days Like This*, the second item in this sequence, is a hiccup, immediately breaking the direction. Simply put, this album is Van at his happiest and poppiest since *Wavelength* seventeen years before, and there in the cover photo, one assumes, is the reason for all this good humour. Making her first appearance on an album cover since Janet Planet adorned the front and back of *Tupelo Honey* is the Morrison Girlfriend. This time, her name was Michelle Rocca, a former Miss Ireland, and the picture shows the happy couple in what seems to be a darkened back alley, walking their matched greyhounds. Ms Rocca's is muzzled.

Perhaps the most striking feature about the album is that, despite all this up-beat poppiness, it contains more songs of complaint than on any previous album: 'Russian Roulette', 'Raincheck', 'Underlying Depression', 'Songwriter' and 'Melancholia' all, at some level, confront Van's demons, and yet still maintain an air of musical insouciance. You have to wonder whether the words of these five songs — or certainly the

A working man in his prime

sentiments that inspired them — date from before Ms Rocca's arrival in Morrison's life, but now that everything is a 'perfect fit', he just can't remain grumpy long enough to give the lyrics the grudging r&b treatment they would normally receive. They're playing russian roulette with your mind? Well, fa la la!

The key to the album is its title track, also the first single, which nicely reverses the imagery in John Lennon's posthumous hit 'Nobody Told Me'. There, Lennon conjures a bizarre world, pitched somewhere between surrealism and satyr, where nothing is right ('Everybody's talking and no one says a word'). Lennon complains that nobody told him 'there'd be days like these', adding parenthetically, 'most peculiar, mama'; in contrast, Morrison seems fully prepared, and, what is more, his 'mama' was the one who told him. Far from the disorientation associated with such days in Lennon's songs, Morrison describes times when everything is going right. Just for once, the bastards are not trying to grind him down and the underlying depression has lifted.

As well as Michelle Rocca, perhaps the choice of Dublin's Windmill Lane Studios as one of the recording locations for *Days Like This* had a positive influence on the singer's mood. He certainly seemed happy enough with the core musicians from the previous album, judging by their appearance here, although Georgie Fame was a notable absentee. Recent additions to the cast of players included singer Brian Kennedy, who'd provided backing vocals on the previous year's live set, and the return of Morrison's horn leader from the late 1970s and early '80s, the great Pee Wee Ellis.

The album kicks off with an up-tempo love song. Simple, breezy and likeable (qualities that made it ideal as the second single off the collection), 'Perfect Fit' includes a line that raises the possibility that 'some people might take the piss' out of the singer's newfound happiness, but it doesn't seem to perturb him. Although the song is couched in the conditional — 'this could be the perfect fit' — we are not left in much doubt that Van believes it. In a coy echo of Karen Carpenter, he tells us they 'haven't even started yet', but he has already worked out that her 'looks' and his 'language' form an irresistible combination. And on the subject of coy echoes, it is on this album that Brian Kennedy's vocals, repeating at the half-bar as much as possible of what Morrison sings, start to become profoundly irritating.

As the title suggests, 'Russian Roulette' draws us into darker and far more complex territory. Is it addressed to the same woman? And if so, is the singer himself now having doubts and trying to remain in control? He insists that 'all this spring fever's just way over my head', which presumably is a reference to being in love. New love is time-consuming, 'stealing my moments' — after all, Van has an album a year to put out. Or two years, as the gaps had been since 1991.

Perhaps she's getting in the way of his songwriting? On this front, 'nothing seems to rhyme', not even that line, which forms a couplet with 'playing Russian Roulette with my mind'. So he has to get away. A visit to Dr John will get his 'mojo working' and then all manner of things will be well. At around this halfway point in the song, the woman he has been addressing is suddenly part of the solution, and no longer the problem. On the contrary, the problem is the 'hustlers', and 'they're playing Russian Roulette with [her] mind', too.

'Raincheck' is a fine song, although reading the lyrics on the page, it is weak, ill-considered and full of clichés.

A working man in his prime

Rhyming 'heart and soul' with 'rock 'n' roll' and 'go, go, go, go, go' is an inauspicious start to any song, while the use of a phrase such as 'need a shot of rhythm and blues' — particularly when it's dissociated from Chuck Berry's original diagnosis of 'rocking pneumonia' — is merely lazy writing. As is often the case, Morrison's poetic diction also becomes a little confused, since he states his intention to 'keep moving on up' while insisting he will also 'stand [his] ground'. But it's a great track nevertheless, partly because of the rather striking line 'My name is raincheck'. Without any further explanation, we know that this is a man who can and does say no, and who, in consequence, runs his own life. Moreover, he 'won't let the bastards grind [him] down'. This, of course, is another cliché, but the music quickly refreshes it. The song is in a gently scampering 6/8, with two beats to the bar, each subdivided into three. But the phrase 'won't let the bastards' is given a bar to itself, with five equal notes, one per syllable. The effect of this 5/8 bar in among all the 6/8 bars is to rush the music, giving it a feeling of urgency and determination, leading naturally to the repeated affirmations ('I don't fade away, unless I choose') that conclude the song. Throughout this performance, which features Arty McGlynn guesting on guitar, Morrison delivers the best singing on the album. Although elsewhere, he is not on top form, distracted even, on 'Raincheck' his flexible vocal ranges impressively from a nimble baritone to a dark growl, everything delivered at great speed.

'You Don't Know Me' is the first of two tracks on the album that are not written by Van Morrison. It seems most likely that Morrison knew this song from Ray Charles's version, and certainly his performance backs up that theory. But its origins as a country-and-western number (it was written by Cindy Walker and Eddy Arnold, and first recorded by Arnold) are underlined by Shana Morrison's additional vocals, and of course this is completely in keeping with a record that bucks the blues/jazz trend of the albums around it.

The contradictions continue in the original material. To hear 'No Religion', for example, is to wonder, momentarily, whether Morrison has finally abandoned his spiritual search altogether. Again, the music is deceptive. The tag line — 'And there's no religion here today' — sounds very pleased with itself, as does the whole song, and it's only on closer inspection of the words that one realises that Van is *unhappy* about the fact there is no religion. He certainly doesn't sound unhappy, and the music's as cheerful here as elsewhere on the album. Indeed, so cloaked in pop pleasantry is 'No Religion' that it was chosen as a third single off *Days Like This*.

The next track, 'Underlying Depression', jogs along nicely, with a fairly standard soul riff on the horns (something like a slowed-down version of the hook on 'Stepping Out Queen' from *Into the Music*, also arranged by Ellis). Morrison's voice is rather fuzzy, as befits his subject here, but this lack of focus is typical enough of his singing on the whole album. At the end, he admits that 'underlying depression ain't nothing but the blues'. So that's all right, then.

On we move to 'Songwriter', yet another complaint song that, on the surface at least, is as cheerful as can be. 'I'm a songwriter,' Van tells us, as though applying for a job, 'and I do it for a living.' The music has a sing-along quality, complete with handclapping on the off-beat. 'Please don't call me a sage,' the singer implores. (So polite!) Still, the rhymes are terrible and the songwriting audition has surely failed.

The title track, with its twist in meaning (Lennon's cliché refreshed), continues the album's positive vibe, and then comes the other non-Morrison song, 'I'll Never Be Free'. Best known in the version by the Red Norvo Quartet, the song was also recorded by Mose Allison, and it is surely this version that inspires Van's. Again with daughter Shana duetting, 'I'll Never Be Free' has a strong country-and-western feel.

Finally, in this sequence of songs, the starkly titled 'Melancholia' does little to bring the mood down. It is slow, certainly, and it makes you want to punch Brian Kennedy, but it isn't any more melancholy than the preceding songs. On the contrary, just as underlying depression has been dismissed as 'nothing but the blues', here we encounter Van 'in the afternoon . . . in my room', coming to terms with a feeling that is 'in my life . . . all the time' by singing about it.

But then the album takes a profound turn. Lyrically, 'Ancient Highway' is one of the many Morrison compendium songs that delivers all the familiar phrases. It's late afternoon (still), the sun is going down, he's in 'a town called Paradise', it's 'near the ancient highway', the train whistle is blowing, the river is flowing, etc. Indeed, the words resemble more of a stream of consciousness than any other Van song since 'You Don't Pull No Punches' back in 1974, and musically there is an equally strong connection. A strummed guitar establishes a harmonically limited palette, over which first a muted trumpet, and later an oboe (Kate St John again), a saxophone and a recorder play slow arabesques, creating a richly multi-layered texture. But the primary layer is provided by Morrison's voice, which, when not free-associating lines from earlier songs about 'a sense of wonder', keeping his 'feet on the ground' and everything being 'right on a Friday evening', is affecting a primal wail through his harmonica. The line that returns most often concerns the singer 'praying to [his] higher self, "Don't let me down"', but there's no specific or literal meaning to the song. Rather, it's Morrison in gruff voice tracing a compelling vocal pattern around snatches of ideas and themes that he's used in countless previous contexts.

'Ancient Highway' seems like the end of the album, but Morrison is not done. Before we go, we return to that scene in his room in the afternoon where 'Melancholia' was set. Singing is one method of dealing with depression, sex is another. 'Wanna make love to you in the afternoon,' Morrison sings. The arrangement is light and laid-back on 'In the Afternoon'. The horns that have contributed so much to the up-tempo feel of the album now play long supporting chords, and gentle punctuating stabs. Morrison's vocals repeat the line 'make love in the afternoon' on and on until, he admits, he is 'talkin' all outta my mind'.

As on *Too Long in Exile*, the healing and spiritual power of sex is made explicit; it can even induce glossolalia. And so an album that began with unbridled happiness and newfound love, ends up with Van and his woman in bed. Of course, Brian Kennedy is there, too, but Van is too outta his mind to care.

In the year that Van Morrison would turn fifty, he had produced one of his rare mainstream pop albums. The words were like no other mainstream pop album, that's for sure, but it was clear from the music that Van the Man was in a very good mood — whatever his latest litany of complaints.

A working man in his prime

THE HEALING GAME
(March 1997)

■ Rough God Goes Riding ■ Fire in the Belly ■ This Weight ■ Waiting Game ■ Piper at the Gates of Dawn ■ Burning Ground ■ It Once Was My Life ■ Sometimes We Cry ■ If You Love Me ■ The Healing Game

As with the comparatively lengthy pause after *Too Long in Exile*, it was nearly two years before Morrison released a follow-up to *Days Like This*. In between came official recognition of his 'services to music', in the form of an OBE, and two more projects that shone light on the singer's roots.

How Long Has This Been Going On was released in December 1995 and was Morrison's 'jazz' album for the Verve label. Recorded live at Ronnie Scott's in London earlier that year, it featured Georgie Fame, who took second billing on the cover, and among the other participants were Van's regular sax players Pee Wee Ellis and Leo Green. With just a handful of Morrison originals among its fourteen tracks, including the previously unreleased 'Heathrow Shuffle', it was a project that did no one any particular credit. On *Tell Me Something: The Songs of Mose Allison*, Morrison was one of four artists given joint billing, the others being Georgie Fame, jazz pianist and producer Ben Sidran and Allison himself. Recorded at what had almost become Van's second home, the Wool Hall, and released in late 1996, *Tell Me Something* topped the US jazz chart, as did the live album.

The Healing Game was Morrison's first album of exclusively original material, since *Enlightenment*, seven years earlier. There on the cover of the disc and in a dozen more photographs inside the booklet is Van, back on the street again with his band. The photography is black-and-white, and the band members are rather sharply dressed in long coats, a hat or two, shirts buttoned up, and even, in the case of horn player Haji Ahkbar, a tie. Van wears dark glasses. In some of the photos, this mainly unsmiling gang seems to be cruising the streets looking for someone who owes them money. On the album cover itself, the side-on angle of Morrison's photograph makes his hat resemble a bowler, while the shiny lapels of his coat suggest a ceremonial sash. For all the world it looks as though Morrison is taking part in an Orange Lodge parade, but it's hard to know whether this was seriously intended.

Surprisingly, given that the singer had spent the whole of the previous decade 'coming home', *The Healing Game* was the first Van Morrison album to be made entirely in Ireland. There, at Dublin's Windmill Lane and Westland studios, he was joined by both his regular band and other musicians with whom he'd recently worked on *How Long* and *Tell Me Something* (pianist Robin Aspland, bassist Alec Dankworth and drummer Ralph Salmins). Also on hand was singer Katie Kissoon.

The album kicks off strongly with 'Rough God Goes Riding', a song about a god which might as well be the Protestant God at His most puritanical and vengeful. When this 'rough god' does as the title states, he leaves a trail of destruction in the form of 'mud-splattered victims', but these victims seem to have been asking for it. They are those

A working man in his prime

who are 'torn between half-truth and victimisation', who throw stones 'in glasshouses', and who leave 'gaping wounds that will never heal'. Given that Van mentions he was 'flabbergasted by the headlines', we can safely assume he's describing the ladies and gentlemen of the tabloid press, who had recently been giving him such a very intrusive time over the Michelle Rocca affair. 'Rough God Goes Riding' is, at one level, Van's revenge fantasy. No wonder he sounds so cheerful; no wonder the music has such a triumphant lilt. No wonder he chose to give the track maximum exposure by releasing it as a single. But the song is more than this, for *The Healing Game* has two central preoccupations, one of which is with presenting contrasting images of god/God, one 'rough', the other benign. The second, related, preoccupation is to do with freeing oneself from different types of negativity and seeking enlightenment.

Next up is 'Fire in the Belly', a song that apparently owes its title to a masculinity self-help book by Sam Keen, purveyor of 'Sex and the Sacred' videos. Morrison employs imagery that goes back to 'A Sense of Wonder', where autumn and spring are 'oh so easy', but 'down through January and February it's a very different thing'. In 'Fire in the Belly', the singer has 'spring' in his heart, a symbol of all his hopes, but before he can reach this goal he's 'gotta get through January . . . gotta get through February'. The music leaves us in no doubt that he will succeed — indeed, the music of *The Healing Game* at all times oozes confidence — but the process will require great reserves of energy and perseverance, and as the album continues, the joyful noise of Morrison's horn-heavy backing band comes to symbolise the transformational power of good, honest (Protestant) hard work.

The burden that Morrison is forced to carry in 'This Weight', is never quite specified, but it seems to be the old problem of fame, and rather than Alice Bailey's illusory 'glamour', the problem this time is the more prosaic matter of tabloid fame. The singer tells us that he desires 'anonymity' and that, in lieu of 'this Hollywood' being 'no good', he wishes (probably because it rhymes) he were 'like Robin Hood'. The most telling lines are towards the end of the song, where he remarks that 'in the very first' he was set free by 'rock 'n' roll', but now 'this weight is just bringing me down'. The track ends with a curious reminiscence of the acappella gospel choir on 'The Eternal Kansas City', from *A Period of Transition*. The band drops out and Morrison, Georgie Fame and Brian Kennedy repeat several more times, unaccompanied, the line 'You know I'm talking 'bout this weight', each time separated by aching silences.

In the next two songs, Morrison is back with images of god. 'Waiting Game' is a curious song and more complex than it first seems. Musically, it feels very pared back after the big-band soul of its predecessors, and a rather dreamy quality pervades. But there's nothing dreamy about a chorus that asserts: 'I am the brother of this snake / I am the serpent filled with venom / A god of love and a god of hate'. What is going on here? The final line appears to argue for the duality of this god (of love and hate), but what of the continual use of the first person? The more one listens, the more one realises that this is a song not so much about god (let alone God), as about Van. The first clue is the use of his stock phrases — it's a 'golden autumn day' and 'the leaves come tumbling down' — but equally, the more one listens, the more we seem to be back in broadly Theosophical/Alice Bailey territory. This god, this 'I', is the 'higher self' to whom Van prayed in 'Ancient Highway' on the previous album, it is 'a presence deep within you'. The duality described in 'Waiting Game' belongs to Morrison's own ego — it is the duality of his 'higher self' — and the waiting game of the song's title is the 'patience' that Morrison must find in order to overcome the 'serpent filled with venom'. So the rather gentle nature of the music is, in the end, entirely fitting. And it leads quite naturally into the rapt stillness of the next track.

'Piper at the Gates of Dawn' is a hymn to Pan, although it has nothing in common with Harrison Birtwistle's wild 'dithyramb' for saxophone and orchestra, *Panic* (or, for that matter, Pink Floyd's debut album of 1967). The starting point for Birtwistle's 1995 piece was the legends of Pan overcoming his enemies by shouting and thereby instilling 'panic' in them. The composer also remembered (as does Morrison) Elizabeth Barrett's poem 'A Musical Instrument', with its image of 'the great god Pan' as a playfully destructive creature: 'Spreading ruin and scattering ban, / Splashing and paddling with hoofs of a goat / And breaking the golden lilies afloat / With the dragon fly on the river'. In Morrison's song we are certainly 'Down in the reeds by the river', but it is the riverbank of Kenneth Grahame's 1908 children's book, *The Wind in the Willows*, and Pan, far from being a 'rough god', is an awesome yet wholly benign presence. The title of Morrison's song, which of course refers to Pan himself, comes from the title that Grahame gave to the central chapter of his book.

On with the show (1992–2003)

The Wind in the Willows is, in part, the story of two creatures, Rat and Mole, and their adventures with and without the famous Toad. In the chapter 'The Piper at the Gates of Dawn', the two friends go in search of a lost baby otter, and the mood of the writing veers radically away from Grahame's rather homely style, the author creating an atmosphere of heady mysticism. As they row along the river, first Rat, then Mole, hears a magical music, issuing, we later learn, from Pan's pipe. It is an illusive sound, no sooner heard than it has vanished, but the memory of it is inextinguishable.

> 'This is the place of my song-dream, the place the music played to me,' whispered the Rat, as if in a trance. 'Here, in this holy place, here if anywhere, surely we shall find Him!'
>
> Then suddenly the Mole felt a great Awe fall upon him, an awe that turned his muscles to water, bowed his head, and rooted his feet to the ground. It was no panic attack — indeed he felt wonderfully at peace and happy — but it was an awe that smote and held him and, without seeing, he knew it could only mean that some august Presence was very, very near. With difficulty he turned to look for his friend, and saw him at his side cowed, stricken, and trembling violently. And still there was utter silence in the populous bird-haunted branches around them; and still the light grew and grew.
>
> Perhaps he would never have dared to raise his eyes, but that, though the piping was now hushed, the call and the summons seemed still dominant and imperious ... Trembling he obeyed, and raised his humble head;

> *and then, in that utter clearness of the imminent dawn, while Nature, flushed with fullness of incredible colour, seemed to hold her breath for the event, he looked in the very eyes of the Friend and Helper . . .*

Grahame's description of Pan stresses the god's benevolence. He has 'kindly eyes', regarding the Rat and the Mole 'humorously, while the bearded mouth broke into a half smile at the corners'. And what's more he has the runaway otter, 'nestling between his very hooves'. In spite of this, though, the animals find themselves trembling in Pan's presence. And eventually,

> *'Rat!' he found breath to whisper, shaking. 'Are you afraid?'*
> *'Afraid?' murmured the Rat, his eyes shining with unutterable love. 'Afraid! Of HIM? Oh, never, never! And yet — and yet — O Mole, I am afraid!'*
> *Then the two animals, crouching to the earth, bowed their heads and did worship,*

It isn't hard to see why this chapter should appeal to Van Morrison. The setting described and the awed tone of the description have featured in many of Morrison's key songs: the woods of 'When Heart Is Open', the autumnal 'days of leaves' of 'A Sense of Wonder', the 'garden wet with rain' of 'In the Garden', and the 'sacred grove' of 'In the Forest'. Morrison's 'Piper at the Gates of Dawn' is almost a paraphrase of Grahame's eponymous chapter. You feel that he must have had the book open beside him as he composed the song. It is dawn, 'they' row the boat on the river, 'they' hear

On with the show (1992–2003)

'the whispering of the reeds' and 'the wind in the willows'. The birds fell silent 'as they listened for the heavenly music'. The music itself (using Grahame's very expression) was a 'song dream', and 'they felt the awe and wonder' on meeting 'the cloven hoofed piper'. If any further proof were needed that Morrison had found in Kenneth Grahame a kindred spirit, it comes as 'they stood upon the lawn and listened to the silence'.

Perhaps because the song is a paraphrase, and because this time the scenario — however uncannily similar to those described in the aforementioned songs — is both second-hand and literary, Morrison's 'Piper at the Gates of Dawn' is not one of his tremulous, awe-struck numbers. There is no attempt at musical transcendence. The song is entirely acoustic, a simple homage to the chapter from Grahame's book, with a rather lovely melody line, and Paddy Moloney showing up just before the end to play two sorts of Irish pipes (first a whistle, then the uillean pipes).

From the bucolic peace of the riverbank, we suddenly lurch into the intense ritual at the heart of *The Healing Game*. The visit to the burning ground was promised way back in 1982 on 'Dweller on the Threshold'. The impatience Morrison described in that song seems to have been overcome (he learned to 'wait', as 'Waiting Game' makes clear) and finally, in this album's 'Burning Ground', the moment has arrived. All that glamour, that heavy 'weight' that Morrison has already sung about, can at last be dumped on 'the burning ground'. The fact that it is referred to as 'the Jute' is potentially mysterious. It is not even clear what sort of jute is meant: is he discussing the hemp-like plant or a resident of

A working man in his prime

Jutland (Denmark)? The printed lyrics accompanying the album use an upper-case J, but that might simply be a matter of attaching import to the ritual. Arguably more significant is the line 'I take the Jute and I throw him down'. *Him*? So this Jute is male?

At one point in her 1922 book *The Gods Await*, Katherine Tingley, the leader of the Theosophical movement for the first quarter of the twentieth century and a well-known prison reformer, described imprisonment as years of being led from a small cell to 'the jute factories' and back. It is possible, then, that Morrison took his image from her book, regarding his unenlightened self as a sort of prisoner, the dumping of 'the Jute on the burning ground' being as good a metaphor as any for his (spiritual) release. But the most probable explanation is the simplest. Sacks are made of jute, and in this sack of woe is 'a ton' of 'glamour'. Wherever the image came from, the meaning, as so often, is clear enough in the performance on the CD, and in the scores of subsequent live performances that would follow. 'Burning Ground' became a regular high point of Morrison's concerts, culminating in the singer either slamming the microphone stand on the ground and jumping up and down on it while screaming 'Stamp on the Jute!', or (possibly after an electrician's intervention) raising the microphone high above his head like a sacrificial offering.

On *Too Long in Exile*, a sequence of three songs — 'Ball & Chain', 'In the Forest' and 'Till We Get the Healing Done' — led to a climax (sexual and spiritual) at the centre of the album that needed a remake of 'Gloria' and a string of other blues numbers to dissipate it. Much the same happens on *The Healing Game*. The burning ground crossed and the Jute duly

On with the show (1992–2003)

dumped, the glamour-free artist can afford to celebrate. The next track, 'It Once Was My Life', looks back at what he has abandoned, which seems mostly to be people who were trying to use him. The lyrics, which oscillate between past and present tense, suggest that he might still need to engage with these people from time to time, but the music — classic, Drifters-style, summer-holiday doo-wop — suggests that he couldn't care less. Let them do their worst! Just bring it on!

'Sometimes We Cry' is another song out of a classic mould. Simple both in diction and musical form, it's a slow, 1950s-style ballad that might have been sung by Buddy Holly or indeed by Johnnie Ray, name-checked here and famous in his time for his inability to get through a stage show without bursting into tears. 'Sometimes we're strong, sometimes we're wrong / Sometime we cry,' Morrison sings. In other words, to everything there is a season: 'Sometimes we live, sometimes we die / Sometimes we cry'. And at least when Van cries, he doesn't 'fake it like Johnnie Ray'. These simple, classic qualities made 'Sometimes We Cry' a perfect candidate for others to cover, and Morrison himself would go on to guest on versions by both Tom Jones, for the latter's *Reload* album in 1999, and daughter Shana three years later. (In fact, all three of these final tracks on *The Healing Game* were soon to be remade with the singer's participation: the next song was Van's contribution to B.B. King's 1997 album of duets, and the title track would be covered this same year by 'the Healer' himself, John Lee Hooker.)

Further evidence of the singer's new-found sanguineness comes on 'If You Love Me'. Now, it seems, he can even take or leave love. It is another doo-wop number underlining his

A working man in his prime

breezy, que sera sera assertion that 'If I love you / I will find the key / If it's meant to be'.

The album's closing track and its first single, 'The Healing Game' itself, is unique. There had been plenty of epic final tracks in three decades of album-making, but nothing so celebratory. It is the culmination of everything else on this remarkably unified album; and it's a hymn of praise, as much, one supposes, to Morrison's 'higher self' and to the process of enlightenment and spiritual healing, as to any god, rough or benign. This time, you feel, the search might really be over. 'Here I am again / Back on the corner again,' Van sings, making a passing reference to one of the Mose Allison songs included on *Tell Me Something*. He tells us he is 'back where I belong' and significantly 'where I've always been'.

It is much as we suspected. Van Morrison has never really been away. Or, to paraphrase T.S. Eliot, he has been off exploring but has now arrived where he started, and finds that he knows the place for the first time. The organ plays, and it is, of course, Georgie Fame's Hammond with its overtones of American gospel and soul, but the rather ruminative chords suggest a church closer to Morrison's childhood, where the organist extemporises as the congregation assembles, and where later 'the choirboys sing'. As Morrison barks out his 'songs of praise' to 'backstreet jellyroll' and to 'the healing game' itself ('Sing it out loud . . . sing it like you're proud'), the horns play, over and over, phrases from Ira Gershwin and Vernon Duke's song: 'I've been around the world in a plane . . . But I can't get started . . .' Morrison, at least for now, has no further need to get started. He has arrived at the beginning. And he knows the place.

On with the show (1992–2003)

BACK ON TOP
(March 1999)

▪ *Goin' Down Geneva* ▪ *Philosopher's Stone* ▪ *In the Midnight* ▪ *Back on Top* ▪ *When the Leaves Come Falling Down* ▪ *High Summer* ▪ *Reminds Me of You* ▪ *New Biography* ▪ *Precious Time* ▪ *Golden Autumn Day*

In June 1998, the long-awaited and long-delayed release of *The Philosopher's Stone* marked a watershed in Van Morrison's career. Having spent the 1980s returning to Ireland, Morrison had devoted most of the 1990s to revisiting his musical roots. In this last pursuit, by 1997, two volumes of greatest hits had appeared, *Too Long in Exile* had included covers of many blues and soul standards, *How Long Has This Been Going On* had been an attempt at jazz, and *Tell Me Something* was a tribute to Mose Allison. 'Gloria' had been re-recorded (in the company of John Lee Hooker), 'Moondance' had been transformed into a big-band number, and *A Night in San Francisco* now rivalled *It's Too Late to Stop Now* as Morrison's greatest live album.

So by 1997, having inspected his roots very thoroughly, Van Morrison knew exactly who he was and so did we. Then, that same year, *The Healing Game* presented Morrison at the end of his spiritual search. All that remained was to put out two rather crowded CDs of previously unreleased material, mainly from the 1970s, which would fill in most of the remaining gaps for his fans, finally allowing us to hear songs such as 'Crazy Jane on God'. And then the story would be complete. But what was Van supposed to do now?

A working man in his prime

The answer to that question was a new album containing more of the same. The archaeological dig through the music of the 1950s and '60s, which commenced in earnest with *Too Long in Exile*, would simply continue. By the end of 2000, the excavations would have uncovered songs as much as half a century old, presented on two further tribute albums, but for now Morrison was happy to keep writing, even if he had nothing to write about.

Yet some changes were in order for the recording of his next album, *Back on Top*, a surprising move given the musical strength of the previous collection. Unlike that Dublin-exclusive project, only this album's strings were recorded at Windmill Lane, the main sessions taking place once again at Wool Hall Studios in Bath. And gone now were almost all of his core musicians stretching back to the *Too Long in Exile* time; the only contributors from *The Healing Game*, in fact, were horn players Pee Wee Ellis and Matt Holland, and Brian Kennedy. The replacements included Mick Green on guitar, and Fiachra Trench, a mainstay over the 1987–91 period, who now returned to play piano as well supplying orchestrations.

Like *The Healing Game*, *Back on Top* contains only Morrison originals, yet each song represented some level of pastiche. For example, 'Goin' Down Geneva', which begins the album, is a driving r&b number with a boogie-woogie piano solo (from Geraint Watkins) and a title that seems to derive from a line in *No Guru*'s 'Foreign Window'; 'Philosopher's Stone' is a classic soul ballad; 'In the Midnight' is a slow doo-wop song, completed by Brian Kennedy's Frankie Valli impersonation. And that's about as much analysis as one needs to give the first four songs on the album.

On with the show (1992–2003)

There are even pastiches of Van Morrison songs. The title track, for example, has our man 'back on the street again' (again) and 'back on top', too, all to the infectious soul-swing familiar from a dozen other Morrison songs. It's high quality, but frankly a bit bland. It might sound like 'These Dreams of You', 'Call Me Up in Dreamland' and 'Kingdom Hall', but it's not as good. And the lyrics are yet another description of how hard it is being famous. Could it be that, by *Back on Top*, Van was really 'not feeling it anymore', as he'd sung on 1991's *Hymns to the Silence*?

'When the Leaves Come Tumbling Down' is a love song that recycles plenty of Morrison's lyric clichés — from the title itself to lines about 'streets in the rain' and even a passing mention of 'the garden' — as well as clichés from other love songs ('the last time I saw Paris'). It has a pretty tune and a certain wistful quality, particularly when you realise that it's a past-tense song, the woman to whom the song is addressed having departed, but by this point in the album, one is beginning to wonder if any of it really matters. The band is as tight and responsive as Van Morrison's bands usually are, and there is no doubt that Van himself is in fine voice, so why is it we find we don't particularly care?

Musically, 'High Summer' is almost a rewrite of 'Dweller on the Threshold', a vital song in the Morrison canon and one that he still regularly sings in concert. But what is this rewrite for? And, more pressingly, what is it about? Notable for the clever hook 'High summer's got him low down' and for its inclusion of the word 'rhododendrons', the lyric can't seem to decide whether it's yet another song about the trials of celebrity or a swift precis of book one of *Paradise Lost*.

A working man in his prime

'Reminds Me of You' is another classic soul ballad — one can almost hear Sam Cooke singing it — and in the context of a better album, it would have made an affecting interlude. The lyrics are a bit corny (everything reminds him of her), but the performance is just fine. It's arguably the strongest song on the album. And then a curious thing happens, almost as if it's a return to the ploy used most effectively on the *No Guru* album: the more one listens, the more Morrison seems to be singing about himself, in this case, singing of his former self. 'I miss you so much when I'm singing my song,' he complains. And so do we.

'New Biography' is very familiar territory, lyrically and musically. There's another doo-wop template for the music, and the lyrics contain a long whinge about his 'so-called friends'. This really is starting to become quite personal, you feel. In the first line of the song, Van notices that 'you've got the new biography' of him, and then explains that he can't see why anyone would be interested in reading it except some sort of loser. You know, the sort of person who is looking for 'a hobby on the internet' (at the last count, the Van Morrison website had nearly three million hits). Morrison singles out those friends who talk to biographers, but by association, he also seems to criticise the sort of person who reads such books. Of course, this is also the sort of person who buys Van Morrison albums and, quite possibly, has been buying them for years, following the seeker on his spiritual search.

Over a bouncy remake of Solomon Burke's 'Gotta Get You Off My Mind', the lyrics of 'Precious Time' make it clear that Morrison has forgotten all about 'the garden': 'It doesn't matter to which God you pray' because we're all going to be

On with the show (1992–2003)

dead shortly. It's now obvious to Van that there's 'no master plan', there's 'no nirvana, no promised land'. So let's dance. Depressing stuff perhaps, but the result was a Top 40 hit in the UK. The other singles, 'Back on Top' and 'Philosopher's Stone', didn't fare so well.

The album's coup de grace is 'Golden Autumn Day', a song that seems, momentarily, as though it will turn out be a classic Morrison number, set as it is among the 'green and pleasant hills' of an Avalon landscape. But then muggers arrive in the car park wielding a knife, before Van, somehow, fights them off, and devotes the remainder of the song to imagining corporal retribution in 'the nearest green field'. One of the most interesting aspects of an exceedingly odd song is its use of the right-wing language of tabloid newspapers. Van's attackers, and others like them, are 'bleeders of the system' and what they need is 'a lesson'. As Fiachra Trench's string ensemble plays its syncopated, pentatonic refrain on the fade — so innocuous! — we are left to contemplate a Van Morrison album that has failed to touch our emotions in any real way, and that has ended with the scourge of the gutter press seeming to join their number.

Is there any satisfactory explanation for *Back on Top*? Perhaps it is the obvious one. The second song on this album, 'Philosopher's Stone', borrows its title and its central image from the 1998 double album of previously unreleased songs. It is a song about songwriting. Just as the philosopher's stone of legend turned base metal into gold, so this songwriter must take unpromising material (and on *Back on Top* some if it is spectacularly unpromising) and make of it a song worth singing.

A working man in his prime

As had been clear for decades, this is not an act that Morrison has much choice about. He is compelled to keep writing songs, whether he wants to or not, and in the past he managed to produce at least a couple of nuggets of gold per album, often many more. The only thing golden on *Back on Top* is the art work.

DOWN THE ROAD
(May 2002)

- Down the Road ■ Meet Me in the Indian Summer ■ Steal My Heart Away ■ Hey Mr DJ ■ Talk Is Cheap ■ Choppin' Wood ■ What Makes the Irish Heart Beat ■ All Work and No Play ■ Whatever Happened to P.J. Proby? ■ The Beauty of the Days Gone By ■ Georgia on My Mind ■ Only a Dream ■ Man Has to Struggle ■ Evening Shadows ■ Fast Train

In 2000, Van Morrison released two CDs, containing a total of twenty-eight songs, only one of which was written by him. The overriding feeling since *Back on Top* was that Morrison, now into his mid fifties, safe in the bosom of Mother Ireland, and with his tortuous spiritual journey seemingly of no importance, had run out of things to write about. The double-header of *The Skiffle Sessions* and *You Win Again* seemed to bear this theory out. It was hard not to feel that, with all due deference to the late, great Lonnie Donegan, Van was made for finer things that a casual saunter through 'Don't You Rock Me, Daddio'.

The Skiffle Sessions was recorded live at Belfast's Whitla Hall over two nights back in November 1998, shortly before

On with the show (1992–2003)

the release of Lonnie's album *Muleskinner Blues*, on which Morrison guested. Van shared the stage with Donegan, band leader Chris Barber and, on two songs, Dr John; Nicky Scott also sat in on bass. To say that it was all a bit of fun is probably overstating the matter. But Donegan obviously enjoyed himself enormously and, one hopes, he died contented the year after the album's release. The material for *The Skiffle Sessions* came, as it had done for the British skiffle bands of the 1950s, from the American folk and country-blues repertoire of Leadbelly, Woody Guthrie, Jimmie Rodgers and others. The songs on *You Win Again*, on the other hand, concentrated more on the country-and-western repertoire of Hank Williams (there are three songs by Williams and more associated with him), together with that single Morrison song, 'No Way, Pedro' (best ignored), and John Lee Hooker's 'Boogie Chillen'. All of it was given an efficient rockabilly treatment, with Linda Gail Lewis standing in on piano for her big brother Jerry Lee, but none of it sounded as though it really needed to be done. One wonders whether Van was simply seeing out his record deal with Virgin.

Morrison released nothing at all the following year, but in 2002 he signed again with Polydor, the company for whom he had made all his albums from *Avalon Sunset* to *The Healing Game*. The association would last for only one album, but it would be an important one.

Back at the Wool Hall (of course), the sessions for this new studio release — his twenty-fifth, and the first in over three years — saw guitarist Mick Green, keyboard players Geraint Watkins and Fiachra Trench, trumpeter Matt Holland and drummer Bobby Irwin retained from the *Back on Top* line-up. Veteran David Hayes returned on bass,

A working man in his prime

having been due a period of long-service leave after serving in two of Van's solo bands; as did John Allair, who'd contributed some keyboards to *Too Long in Exile* but otherwise had been off the rollcall since 1984. Colin Griffin, Pete Hurley and Lee Goodall, on drums, bass and saxophone respectively, were newly recruited from the collaboration with Linda Gail Lewis.

Down the Road made its intentions very clear even before the listener got it to the CD player. The cover showed a shop window full of old LP sleeves, including images of all the figures whose songs Morrison had been singing for the past decade: Ray Charles, Mose Allison, Leadbelly, Hank Williams and the rest. But was the new album just going to be more of the same, only this time with a classy cover?

The title track, up first, makes it immediately clear that one of those 'returns to form' is on the cards. It is obvious from the first minute that Morrison's music has become honest again. All that ridiculous posturing of *Back on Top* has gone. Now we find a lonely man, forced to keep going 'down the road' by his need to create new songs. These songs will always come out in certain ways because of his make-up and because of his memories. He has the blues 'from way down in New Orleans', and he admits that the 'memories, dreams and reflections' of great music, there for all to see on the cover of the record, 'keep haunting' him. He must respond to the call of 'those gypsy voices' but he is only capable of responding in certain ways. The fact that the music strides out in a confident, carefree G major, suggests that in addition to facing up to his responsibilities and limitations as a songwriter, he also accepts them. This is frankly encouraging.

On with the show (1992–2003)

'Meet Me in the Indian Summer' is an up-tempo, feel-good soul number, with plenty of horn solos. Where on the previous album's 'Golden Autumn Day' Morrison was 'taking in the Indian summer' and merely 'pretending that it's paradise', the Indian summer of *Down the Road* seems like a fine place, 'not bound by any definition' and a good jumping-off point for 'eternity'. At first, it doesn't appear to be a terribly profound song, but the more one thinks about a pop-music figure of Morrison's generation and stature, singing about the Indian summer of his life and happily acquiescing in it instead of railing at the world (as he had on *Back on Top*), the more impressive it becomes. He is content where he is and invites us to join him there.

So, having headed off 'down the road' with equanimity and arranged to meet us in the 'Indian summer' thence to 'go walking to eternity', Morrison admits, on track three, that 'the journey's longer than I thought'. Perhaps he's simply surprised to discover that he can still fall in love. At any rate, 'Steal My Heart Away' is a love ballad set to a tripping waltz metre, and this time Van is promising his love that he will come to her 'just like the sunshine after rain'; and while he's there again she will 'steal [his] heart away'.

As in the second half of *The Healing Game*, on this album Morrison is taking simple musical forms (the straight-ahead soul celebration, the slow waltz) and pouring rather simple thoughts into them. The next song is actually on the subject of the potency of such simple music, to paraphrase Noël Coward.

'Hey Mr DJ', which itself was the first single taken from *Down the Road*, is a song about singles. Addressed to a disc jockey — the old-fashioned sort of DJ, who just used to play other people's records — it's is a request for a familiar song ('something that I know'), the sort of song that, on account of its familiarity, will cheer us up right from the opening chords. Because 'Hey Mr DJ' is about familiarity, it needs to sound familiar, and it does. The loping bass, the saxophone and the strings immediately suggest the world of Sam Cooke (a song such as 'Wonderful World'), so that 'Hey Mr DJ' ends up satisfying its own request.

Now the songs begin to come thick and fast. 'Talk Is Cheap' is a classic Morrison song of complaint, delivered (since this is a traditional album) as a twelve-bar blues, but with a new note of reasonableness in its final line. Yes, tabloid newspapers are terrible things, full of 'backbiters and syndicators', and anyone who talks to them is a 'goddamn fool', but finally Morrison concedes that 'talk is cheap *almost* all the time'. And that is quite a concession.

On 'Choppin' Wood', another blues, Van tells the story of his father's journey to the United States in search of work. He failed and returned from Detroit but he had done the best he could and 'kept on choppin' wood'. Rather than the meditative associations it carried in 'Enlightenment', the wood-chopping metaphor now seems a straightforward reference to repetitive work, or perhaps to the Protestant work ethic. At any rate, we're a long way from Zen.

Despite its Foster and Allen title, 'What Makes the Irish Heart Beat' is an interesting song dealing with Morrison's own absence from Ireland. Although the song has a strong country-and-western flavour, this absence was not when he was in America, but in London, and specifically under an

On with the show (1992–2003)

advertisement for Wrigley's chewing gum at Piccadilly Circus. The opening lines suggest that the singer was driven from Belfast by the Troubles, but this seems doubtful. Sectarian violence in Ulster didn't really escalate until the late 1960s, by which time Morrison had been living in the United States for at least a year. So, 'All that trouble, all that grief / That's why I had to leave' must either be a reference to something else altogether in his life or just a good couplet he didn't want to waste.

'All Work and No Play', the next track, is yet another twelve-bar blues. It's as playful as its title suggests, with a cornucopia of horn solos, including one from Van himself that may well be the best he has ever achieved in this department, at least in the studio. The high spirits of the song turn, just before the end, into the Duke Ellington Orchestra's 'Things Ain't What They Used to Be', and this playful postmodern referencing continues into the final number of this six-song sequence at the centre of the album.

It's Ray Charles's 'Hit the Road Jack' that is unmistakeably invoked as the introduction to 'Whatever Happened to P.J. Proby?' Of course, on one level, the thought of 'the road' is meant to take us back to the album's title — this is a carefully laid-out affair — but it also reminds us of the road down which we walk 'to eternity' in 'Meet Me in the Indian Summer'. And whatever *did* happen to P.J. Proby? Proby was an impressive and hugely charismatic rock and soul performer from America who exploded into the British pop scene in the mid 1960s, while the rest of the world had its eyes and ears focused on the music coming *out* of Britain. In fact, he almost literally exploded. Blame it on the tight velvet pants. There came a moment in his stage show when the seam at the front couldn't take it anymore and, to the great delight of the girls in the front row (and the consternation of their parents when they heard about it on the news), the pants split. For this reason, if no other, his success in Britain was meteoric, and after 1965 he was scarcely heard of again, prompting Van Morrison's very pertinent query. But the most important question in what might at first pass for a novelty song is in the final line: 'And whatever happened to me?'. The suggestion here is that nothing is what it was (which is incontestable), and furthermore that nothing is as good as it was (which could be hotly debated). But Morrison's question is also rhetorical, for he knows perfectly well what happened to him. Other performers of the 1960s might have become mere websites of their former selves, but Morrison, like his father, 'kept on choppin' wood'.

On 'The Beauty of the Days Gone By', Morrison hymns the past, and it's a suitably stylised, indeed sentimentalised past, complete with a 'mountain glen where we used to roam'. The word 'roam' alerts us to this sentimentality. There is something self-consciously poetic about it (as there is with 'doth' in the previous verse) and this tends to undercut the assertion 'Oh my memory, it does not lie'. Of course it does — everybody's memory lies, we are prone to sentimentalise the past. But if, as the singer suggests two songs later, our lives are 'only a dream', then what does the unreliability of memory matter? Morrison's past and particularly his childhood have been his inspiration ever since *Astral Weeks*, and not surprisingly his despised biographers have tended to concentrate their efforts on these years in order to explain the nature of this inspiration. It is not

On with the show (1992–2003)

without value, this search, but it should always be remembered that Van Morrison's songs are built in his imagination, and, like everyone else's imagination, that is influenced by memory. Far more significant for Morrison's work than the precise details of his early life are his memories of viaducts and pylons and Ray Charles singing 'I Believe to My Soul', of 'the days of leaves', 'streets wet with rain' and 'the mountain glen where we used to roam'.

Appropriately, 'The Beauty of the Days Gone By' is separated from 'Only a Dream' by the album's only cover, a song that, thanks to Ray Charles, would have been popular in Morrison's youth. Indeed, it is very much Charles's version of 'Georgia on My Mind' that Morrison is busy adding tropes to here, and the song's composer, Hoagy Carmichael, would barely recognise this account.

Way back on *Moondance*, 'Ray Charles was shot down' in a dream Morrison had, but in 'Only a Dream' it is Van who's 'knocked ... off [his] feet' while 'somebody' attempts to knock the dream itself down. And all the while 'the big band kept on playing, of "Bonaparte's Retreat"', which is another song from Morrison's childhood, a hit for Kay Starr (who also scored with 'The Lonesome Road', a cover of which appears on *Too Long in Exile*). In the original song, a man takes his girl in his arms and kisses her 'while the fiddles played "The Bonaparte's Retreat"', and now, in Morrison's song, a band is performing the song. This is more than Van taking us back once more to his fabled childhood; we are at some church-hall dance with a show band, and this image, you suddenly realise, is the key to the whole album. Van has taken us back this time to his early professional roots. The range of songs, the range of styles, and the breezy, brassy treatment meted out to them: all this suggests the essential versatility of a show band, albeit in this case a particularly classy one.

And right on cue, here comes Acker Bilk, clarinettist, composer and band leader who made his Paramount Jazz Band into one of the classiest acts of the singer's youth. (Although, for reasons best known to his record company no doubt, European CD buyers were treated to the truly terrible 'Man Has to Struggle' straight after 'Only a Dream', a pointless insertion that interferes with the album's logical sequencing.) 'Evening Shadows' is a Bilk tune fitted out with words by Morrison and turned into a surprisingly cheery number about lost love, in which, by the by, Morrison is once more 'living in a dream'.

At the end of every show-band set comes the inevitable slow dance, and this set is no exception. Contrary to its title, 'Fast Train' is a slow song, and by putting it at the end of *Down the Road*, Van Morrison is bringing us and, doubtless, himself back down to earth. This 'fast train' is an illusion, because it's 'going nowhere'. It is also a metaphor for a relationship, one that is 'going off the rails'. But who is the other party in this relationship? Is it us, the listeners? 'Fast Train' is a complex song, one that not only brings to an end the musical variety show we've experienced, but also brings us full circle (the image of 'going nowhere' is appropriate in that sense, too). An album that had begun with the singer heading off 'down the road' to do his job (to write songs and sing them for us) — and to do this because he must, because that's what singers do — concludes with a song about more journeys to be undertaken. He must go 'on the lam', and the journey will be tough. One moment there is 'sleet and snow' out there, then the journey involves travelling 'across the desert sand, through the barren waste'. But everywhere are images of breakdowns, and this traveller is on his own. No one's on his 'waveband', and there is no 'helping hand'. The point is that he is doing all this partly for us. The song — the entire album — is an offering, an apology, if you like, after the sheer rudeness of *Back on Top*.

But it is not simply that Morrison has realised that he owes this to his loyal supporters. Something more fundamental and more important is happening. *Back on Top* wasn't just churlish, it was self-deluding; it was an attempt to deny what he had learned on *The Healing Game*. *Down the Road*, a little reluctantly, a little wearily, accepts the truth. All Van Morrison can do is keep on writing songs and singing them. He must keep on going 'down the road', climbing on that fast rain, even when it's off the rails. Like his dad, he has to keep on 'choppin' wood'.

WHAT'S WRONG WITH THIS PICTURE?
(October 2003)

- *What's Wrong With This Picture?* ■ *Whinin' Boy Moan*
- *Evening in June* ■ *Too Many Myths* ■ *Somerset* ■ *Meaning of Loneliness* ■ *Stop Drinking* ■ *Goldfish Bowl* ■ *Once in a Blue Moon* ■ *Saint James Infirmary* ■ *Little Village* ■ *Fame*
- *Get on with the Show*

Van Morrison's first album for Blue Note, his third record label in as many releases, was notable for the glorious sound of his voice. It was cleaner and more focused than of late and the man himself sounded about thirty years younger. That is not to say he sounded as he did in 1973 on *It's Too Late to Stop Now*, rather that he seemed like a *different* much younger man. Whatever the reason for this — vitamins? filters? — the effect on the music was energising. And on the title track, at the start of the second verse, he actually bursts out laughing.

Something good must have been going on, then, during the sessions for *What's Wrong With This Picture?* and pleasingly, given the return to form of his previous CD, a good many of the musicians from *Down the Road* were also in attendance this time around, as were some other familiar faces. On guitars were Ned Edwards (from *You Win Again*, the collaboration with Linda Gail Lewis) and Foggy Lytle (who'd played on 1995's *Days Like This*), and the previous album's Mick Green and Johnny Scott; Richard Dunn and Fiachra Trench returned on keyboards, while new in was Gavin Povey; bass duties were shared by David Hayes and Pete Hurley once more, and Nicky Scott, now back in the fold; drummer Bobby Irwin was there yet again, alternating with Liam Bradley (another who'd appeared on *Days Like This*, and *Back on Top*); Alan 'Sticky' Wickett played percussion (as he'd done back at the Whitla Hall in '98 for *The Skiffle Sessions*); and as before, horns and reeds were in the capable hands of Lee Goodall, Matt Holland, Martin Winning and special guest Acker Bilk, joined on the title track by Keith Donald on bass clarinet.

The laughter on 'What's Wrong With This Picture?', the opening song, might have been spontaneous, though to be honest it doesn't really sound it. But even if it was planned down to the last chuckle, the sound of the creator of *Back on Top* laughing (note, not sneering) two minutes into his new album comes as a small revelation. And then there's the string orchestra mooching its way through a verse of the song before Van even opens his mouth. So what *is* wrong with this picture?

Well, on the face of it, not very much at all. Having realised on *Down the Road* that he was, above all, the leader of a show band, on *What's Wrong With This Picture?* Morrison sets out to prove it and, in the words of the final track, to 'get on with the show'. From its quietly arresting opening, the first song leads us into the gentle reaches of a Ray Charles–like ballad. The words are all about Van not being 'that person anymore', he has left 'all that jive behind'. The world is an unreliable place; 'you can't believe what you read in the newspapers' and TV is no better. He's moving on. That picture 'hanging on a wall' — that's who he 'used to be'. And *that's* what's wrong with it. Let's 'take it down', he suggests. We've heard all this before, of course, but the curious thing now, at least for anyone who is not a Morrison neophyte, is that the words have simply ceased to matter. It's the music that counts.

From the ballad, we plunge headlong into a bar-room blues. The coin goes into the jukebox and the band pumps away. 'Whinin' Boy Moan' takes its title from an old Jelly Roll Morton song, and Morton himself is mentioned again as 'Mr Jelly Roll', the title of Alan Lomax's biography. Like most of this singer/pianist's oeuvre, 'The Whinin' Boy' stressed Morton's masculinity and his availability as a sexual surrogate. Given that Morrison's song is about letting the 'whinin' boy moan if you don't know how to do it yourself', it would seem to be on a topic very close to Morton's original, and some of Morrison's imagery might need to be reconsidered in that light — beginning in the first line with that coin going 'right into the

A working man in his prime

slot'. Like 'What's Wrong With This Picture?', 'Whinin' Boy Moan' employs stock-standard lyrics in the service of giving Morrison's voice a good workout. And he doesn't disappoint. It's hard to think when he last produced such a party of a song, his vocals almost jitterbugging through the track.

The lyrics of 'Evening in June', which ends its first line with the word 'moon' and includes references to 'a sleepy lagoon' (thank you, Harry James) and the 'flowers ... in bloom', could scarcely be more stock. And Morrison surely knows it. He might be as instinctive a songwriter as he is a singer, but even the least self-demanding writer knows you can't make a rhyme out of 'moon' and 'June' with a straight face. A pattern is emerging: 'Evening in June' is a classic pop song, in inverted commas, just as 'Whinin' Boy Moan' is a blues-in-quotes and 'What's Wrong With This Picture?' is not a genuine Ray Charles ballad. It isn't that the songs are a series of fakes. On the contrary, 'Evening in June' has a catchy melody — something that isn't exactly common in Morrison's work — and it is particularly well sung, Van's voice becoming clearer and truer the longer the album continues. No, what we are listening to is another show-band set. Van's band on this album is not unlike the Beatles' idea of turning themselves into Sgt Pepper's Lonely Hearts Club Band for an album. The band on *What's Wrong With This Picture?*, even more so than on *Down the Road*, is a show band putting itself through its paces and demonstrating its versatility. There might be a large dose of banality in the material but, as he explained on 'Philosopher's Stone' on *Back on Top*, it's a matter of turning lead into gold, and by and large here the performances do that.

On with the show (1992–2003)

So, after 'Too Many Myths', a blues about how you're only as good as your last gig ('I got my name up in lights / But I've still gotta keep my game uptight'), it's time to welcome back Mr Acker Bilk for another guest spot, on 'Somerset'. As on the previous album's 'Evening Shadows', the West Countryman again brings an old hit to which Morrison has supplied the words. The structure of the album, it is true, rather closely resembles that of *Down the Road*, but the music is bolder and the performances much stronger. If it's more of the same, then, who cares?

'Meaning of Loneliness' is a fine song about depression — indeed about 'existential dread' — and for the first time in a decade (unless you count the passing reference to Blake on 'Golden Autumn Day' from *Back on Top*), Morrison mentions some literary figures. Dante is there as part of a joke, but when Van gets down to the serious stuff about 'the meaning of loneliness', he mentions Sartre and Camus as though he has done some of the right reading on the subject; and then for good measure he throws in Nietzsche and Hesse (both of whose names he mispronounces).

'Stop Drinking' is a Lightnin' Hopkins song, fitted out with a whole new set of clothes, and a few new words, when Morrison turns it into a rockabilly number — and a particularly lively one at that. This partly undermines the sermon he is about to deliver on the subject of not being a rock singer, but it doesn't deter him.

After an album and a half of show-band behaviour, and in the guise of a slow, Chicago-style blues, 'Goldfish Bowl' sees Van pausing to explain precisely what it is that he's up to. There are two parts to this. First, he is not famous, let that be understood. No hit record, no TV show: why would anybody possibly be interested in him? Second, and really more important, is the fact that he sings 'jazz, blues and funk' as well as 'folk with a beat and a little bit of soul', none of which is anything remotely like rock 'n' roll. Now is that clear?

The next song is a rarity in every sense. 'Once in a Blue Moon' is not jazz, blues or funk or any of the other categories he has just been insisting he is wedded to. Its general musical style seems to emanate from somewhere in the Caribbean — say, a Trinidadian resort particularly favoured by holidaying Mariachi bands. It is up-tempo, the most thoroughly cheerful Morrison song since 'Perfect Fit' eight years before, and it is hard to understand why it failed to become a hit when released as a single, except that it would seem to be a point of honour for Morrison that he has 'no hit record'.

On that great blues 'Saint James Infirmary', forever associated with the trumpet of Louis Armstrong, the show band abruptly swaps its sombreros for the more dignified garb of a New Orleans funeral procession. But anyone expecting the customary 'Second Line' jazz celebration that traditionally follows such an occasion will be surprised by the Dylanesque guitar thrumming that leads into the ensuing track.

'Little Village', a twelve-bar blues without any blues chords, describes an idyll in a mountain village. It features not only 'long cool summer nights' but bells, moonlight through trees, a forest wet with rain, and even 'the voice of silence'. As on *Down the Road*, the passing cavalcade of musical styles has found room for a 'Van Morrison' song. And as though to underline the point, 'Little Village' is followed by a different sort of Morrison number, 'Fame', a belly-aching blues on the

On with the show (1992–2003)

subject of 'fame' and how 'they' (the newspapers again?) have 'taken everything and twisted it'.

'Get on with the Show' (sound advice under the circumstances) is a catchy, Sam Cooke-style song, with an amusing middle eight about Nero and Napoleon, Samson and Delilah, and David and Goliath, some strident sax solos and a little vintage Morrison barking among some otherwise very clean and straight singing by the born-again baritone. There's a wry nonchalance about this most toe-tapping of finales, as though Morrison can't help remembering the final tracks of some of his other albums: 'Slim Slow Slider', 'Almost Independence Day', 'You Know What They're Writing About', 'When Heart Is Open'. 'I just wanna get on with the show,' he insists. 'And if it don't work then let it go.'

At the end of *What's Wrong With This Picture?*, you can't help but feel Morrison has been reunited with his first show band, only they've had more than four decades to practice. Van Morrison has been many things during his long career, but on this album he is purely an entertainer. The spiritual searcher seems content, the grumpy businessman at least partially reconciled to his lot, and the bandleader and singer appears suddenly in his prime.

Was this, after all, what Morrison was searching for? Was his goal always, in fact, spiritual in the Protestant sense of reward for hard work? Is this — the pub, the community centre, the town hall, the nightclub, any stage in any town — the beginning at which Morrison has wanted to arrive? The only possible answer to these questions is a new album.

EPILOGUE

SPEAKING IN TONGUES: THE VOICE OF VAN MORRISON

'Tura . . . lura . . . lural,' sings Richard Manuel from the stage of San Francisco's Winterland on Thanksgiving Day 1976. 'Tura . . . lura . . . lye . . .' At first the crowd is amused, then a little mystified. This is the Band's final concert — why is Manuel singing a *lullaby*?

'Tura . . . lura . . . lural,' he repeats, drawing out the words as before. '*Hush* . . . don't you cry.' The audience dutifully quietens down.

By the time the piano player has sung the third line, a few people in the crowd are beginning to get it; they've worked out the identity of the next guest. Spontaneous smatterings of applause are breaking out.

Epilogue

'Tura ... lura ... lural,' Manuel sings one last time, the applause spreading around the hall. 'That's an *Irish* lullaby ...' Gradually the crowd begins a roar of approval, and out on stage walks the Belfast Cowboy, Van the Man.

Lullabies have a dual function in the lives of parents and children, their words and music seldom matching. Commonly enough, the words are rather violent, relating stories of babies falling from treetops (in 'Rock-a-bye Baby') or innocent fluffy lambs having their eyes pecked out ('All the Pretty Little Horses'). Some writers have pointed to a superstitious rationale for this. The horrors are conjured up so as to ward off actual danger; as Marina Warner has put it, by naming untold disasters in the nick of time, the singer of the lullaby ensures that those same dangers are less likely to strike the child. More credible, perhaps, is the theory that lullabies belong to a musical genre that also includes cotton-picking songs and sea shanties: in other words, they are work songs for mothers. As with all such songs, the musical metre (in this case a lulling 6/8) assists with the work — the rocking of a cradle — while the words, in common with all work songs, abuse or even threaten the taskmaster. And in this case the taskmaster is the baby. Since the baby cannot understand the words, lullabies can be about anything at all. They can even be nonsense ('Tura lura lural'). What the child identifies with above all in this process — and what, in consequence, gets the job done and the child to sleep — is the sound of the mother's voice, soothing in its familiarity. 'In singing,' writes Mark W. Booth in *The Experience of Songs*, 'whatever version of motherhood the words express, the mother's voice is especially motherly'.

Epilogue

Whether Van Morrison is singing an Irish traditional song, a soul standard or the blues, or a song of his own in any of the above styles or combinations of them — or, for that matter, a lullaby — his listeners, and particularly his fans, will be first and foremost aware of the sound of his voice. It is hard to overstate the importance of that vocal familiarity in Morrison's enduring appeal. Among his contemporaries and peers, there are few such familiar sounds and fewer familiar voices. Bob Dylan's harmonica would surely count as a sound of equal familiarity. Dylan's voice, of course, is also hugely distinctive, but it hasn't remained constant. The harmonica playing, however, always a triumph of brute force over technique and good taste, has retained its singularity, Dylan's refusal to give up on the instrument making a virtue of his seemingly random sucking and blowing. And even today, when that first harmonica note wails in concert, the audience always cheers. They recognise a sound they have known, in many cases, all their lives.

Another example of instant recognition is Miles Davis's trumpet. Either unadorned or with its Harmon mute inserted but the stem removed, the instrument's timbre was unmistakeable, and it shared with Morrison's singing voice a stylistic flexibility. Davis's trumpet wandered freely from the Gil Evans Orchestra to the quintet with Coltrane, to the one with Wayne Shorter, to the glittering electric baubles of *Bitches Brew*, to the hard-rocking band of the *Jack Johnson* sessions, finally coming to rest in a funky world of 'modern standards' playing tunes by Cyndi Lauper and Michael Jackson. But the sound was always itself.

Morrison's voice can do many things. It can moan and shout, produce short staccato barks and long inner growls; it can caress and wheedle and keen. But it too is always itself. With the possible exception of the edgy falsetto that he seems to have given up sometime in the late 1970s, and which is therefore perhaps unfamiliar to more recent converts, there are no versions of this voice that his fans would fail to recognise. The meaning of Van's songs is in his voice, and when he abandons words completely, the meaning goes deepest.

One vocal tradition to which Morrison's wordless singing is strongly related isn't really a musical tradition at all. Charismatic Christians might commence their acts of worship from a prayerbook or a hymn sheet (in the beginning, after all, was the Word), but the high point of religious ecstasy comes when text is transcended, the spirit fills the worshipper and speaking in tongues ensues. Morrison himself sings songs in many tongues — from the Chicago blues to Irish folk songs, from jazz, to soul, to rock 'n' roll — but in live performance the call-and-response patterns frequently established with a band member or backing vocalist strongly suggest the influence not only of gospel music, but of the Pentecostal church. At a linguistic level, Pentecostal glossolalia is semantic twaddle, but it is anything but meaningless to the believer. When Van is muttering the word 'viaduct' to himself, over and over, or shouting triumphantly about stamping 'on the Jute', there is meaning there too. We might not understand it, but we certainly feel it.

There are examples of wordless singing in most cultures, and in very many of them the absence or abandonment of words implies an elevated state. At the very least, it betokens a kind of emotional honesty, as Peter Conrad proposes in *A Song of Love and Death: The Meaning of Opera*:

Epilogue

Love and hate tend to reduce us to speechlessness — to embarrassed stammering, or to expletives ... Words are always failing us when we need them most. To remain articulate in states of extreme emotional intensity almost convicts us of insincerity. Love poetry often apologises for its linguistic fluency, afraid it will seem specious. But when words give up, music takes over.

On a good night, the music always takes over with Morrison, and he begins to use his voice like an instrument. Even when he is singing words, which is most of the time, the way he sings them is far and away more important than the words themselves. This is not intended to suggest that his lyrics are insignificant or short on meaning (although sometimes they are), but that more often than not the significance is greatly enhanced and the meaning clarified by the manner of his vocal delivery. This explains why, at least compared to those of Bob Dylan, Morrison's songs have been rarely recorded by others: divorced from the songwriter's own performance, the material is nearly always less impressive and often banal. It also explains why Morrison's success at singing other peoples' songs is variable: those songs that demand a blues/soul delivery and performances that elevate style above substance (including, for example, all the cover versions on *It's Too Late to Stop Now*) nearly always come off, whereas those that require careful and detailed attention to convoluted lyrics (Ira Gershwin's 'How Long Has This Been Going On?', say, or W.B. Yeats's 'Crazy Jane on God') seldom seem worth the singer's effort. Standing in Ronnie Scott's club in June 1986

Epilogue

alongside the Chet Baker Trio, Morrison attempts Stephen Sondheim's 'Send in the Clowns'. He reads from a piece of paper, which presumably bears Sondheim's lyrics, but he still manages to fluff the words. When occasionally his own songs have complex lyrics — 'Rave on, John Donne', for instance — these too can trip him up: 'Oh what swine . . . sweet *wine* we drink . . .', he stammers on *Live at the Grand Opera House, Belfast*.

Words are not really Van Morrison's metier, not in the literary sense. He is not a poet like Dylan, however much his name might be linked to Blake and Yeats, and however often he might pose the question 'Did you ever hear about Wordsworth and Coleridge, baby?'. Unlike those of Dylan, Lennon and McCartney, Lou Reed or Joni Mitchell, Morrison's lyrics have not and surely will not be anthologised. In Van's songs, the words have two basic functions. First, they quickly tell the listener what sort of song it is: a 'cool, clear crystal water' song or a 'backstreet jellyroll' song or a 'piss off and leave me alone' song. Second, they provide a structure for Morrison's singing, a platform from which, if we are lucky, he might launch into one of his extended and wordless vocalisations. These are the moments that devotees of Van the Man wait for. When the sound of his voice usurps the performance, when words fly out the window, when a state of musical rapture descends on the singer, and the song he was singing becomes just a memory; when moaning, growling and keening take over or, out of the rubble of the lyrics, some word or phrase is salvaged and repeated, mantra-like, in a nasal whine or a rasping whisper. This is Morrison performing a kind of instrumental with his voice.

Epilogue

In the 1980s, Morrison recorded a surprising number of genuinely instrumental tracks. Specifically, from 1982 to 1987, on the albums *Beautiful Vision*, *Inarticulate Speech of the Heart*, *A Sense of Wonder* and *Poetic Champions Compose*, he included no fewer than nine instrumentals, variously playing piano, guitar and saxophone. Some of these were exceptionally bland — one thinks in particular of 'Scandinavia', the final track on *Beautiful Vision* — and in all of them, Morrison's rather basic playing skills contributed to the lack of excitement. The keyboard technique required to play the solo on 'Scandinavia', utilising only the black keys, could be taught to a reasonably musical person with no previous experience of the piano in about ten minutes. The same technique (and more or less the same riffs) turn up on 'Inarticulate Speech of the Heart No. 1' and again on 'Evening Meditation' from *A Sense of Wonder*, although now the playing is limited to the white keys.

On 'Boffyflow and Spike', also from *A Sense of Wonder*, Morrison had Ireland's crack folk band Moving Hearts to give his music a significant lift, but even they could not save this rather earthbound melody. By 1987 and the release of *Poetic Champions*, an album that begins with a five-minute instrumental, his saxophone playing had certainly improved, but the fact remains that nobody has ever bought a Van Morrison album for the instrumentals. And if you're going to listen to three saxophone solos lasting nearly a quarter of an hour, you would hope they might be played by Lee Konitz or Joe Lovano.

But the musical contents of these instrumentals, although unexceptional, are worth examining because they form such a

Epilogue

contrast to Morrison's wordless 'instrumentals'. 'Boffyflow and Spike' is an attempt at a traditional Irish reel (and fittingly, Van would re-record it with the Chieftains for their 1989 album *Chieftains Celebration*); it's ineluctably fake, but pleasant enough in a toe-tapping kind of way. 'Spanish Steps', the opening track of *Poetic Champions*, is an uncredited reworking of the slow movement of Joaquín Rodrigo's *Concierto de Aranjuez* filtered through Miles Davis and Gil Evans's earlier reworking on *Sketches of Spain*. Those aside, there is a lot of that pentatonic doodling à la 'Scandinavia'.

Yet two tracks stand out among these instrumentals, and that is because on them Morrison's solo instrument is his own voice. These are 'September Night', the final item on *Inarticulate Speech of the Heart* (and as one listens to it, the album's title takes on a new significance), and 'Evening Meditation'. The latter, as mentioned, is aimless in its white-note pentatonicism, and yet the piano, organ and the singer's wordless voice fuse into a strangely powerful unison that lends distinction to an otherwise workaday melodic line. 'September Night' is a different matter. Harmonically it is subtler, and the main melodic line is sung (wordlessly) by a small group of female vocalists. Morrison's vocal contribution is limited to interjections pitched somewhere between the sound of a muted trumpet and a horse's whinnying. Again, it is his voice that makes the difference, creating something strange, emotional and slightly disturbing out of a gently pleasing melody.

Far better examples of the power of Morrison's voice come in those songs in which lyrics are first sung, and then either abandoned or repeated such that they lose their meaning. While

Epilogue

this might have been happening ever since *Astral Weeks* ('To love to loves to love to loves . . .' etc.), with a later example being the nasal keening at the end of *Irish Heartbeat*'s 'She Moved Through the Fair', it was on *Common One* that it reached epic proportions. 'Summertime in England' has already been discussed as one of the key Morrison songs, but 'When Heart Is Open' is its almost wordless complement. Together they occupy more than half an hour of the album.

'When Heart Is Open' is a song without harmony and without tempo. Specifically, this piece of music sits for its entire duration above a drone (the note E), while various melodic strands — Mark Isham's trumpet, Pee Wee Ellis's flute, Van's voice, with and without harmonica — tug at it like a sitar player in an classical Indian raga. Closer to home, and perhaps more pertinently, the influence of Miles Davis can be heard in this track. The timbre of Isham's trumpet is immediately reminiscent of Davis, and the ambience of the song strongly suggests close acquaintance with albums such as *In a Silent Way* and *Bitches Brew*. Like much of that music (and again like the *alap* of a raga), the apparently spontaneous melodic phrases and fragments of phrases in 'When Heart Is Open' create localised tempi, animating the surface of the music. But without exception, these moments are fleeting. To all intents and purposes, this music is static.

So 'When Heart Is Open' is a significant and unique moment in Morrison's output. But is it not also contrived? Van's vocal cadenza just before the end is beautifully judged, but it does not sound especially 'heartfelt'. There is no loss being wailed over here; on the contrary, the singer sounds very

Epilogue

comfortable and, when compared to his work on a song such as 'Listen to the Lion', even a bit smug. In the version on *Saint Dominic's Preview* and the live account on *It's Too Late to Stop Now*, the power of 'Listen to the Lion' is that of a simple strophic song which collapses on itself. 'Things fall apart,' Yeats wrote in 'The Second Coming', 'the centre cannot hold.' What is lost, at least temporarily, in 'Listen to the Lion' is the song itself, and Morrison's wailing for this loss, his keening and roaring, are performed in defiance of Yeats's 'mere anarchy'.

In *A Song of Love and Death*, Conrad advances the theory that opera is 'drama about music, not just accompanied by it'. For this reason, singers can and regularly do dispense with words, examples ranging from Lucia and her 'crazed conversation with a flute' in the famous mad scene from Donizetti's *Lucia di Lammermoor*, to Mozart's Queen of the Night losing her cool and, in her fury, scat-singing those high Fs in *The Magic Flute*. It is not drawing such a very long bow to suggest that Van Morrison's songs, for all their stated and implied themes as discussed in this book, are also really 'about music' and, more specifically, about the power of the voice. On the surface, the words might seem to tell other stories, stories of home (leaving home, finding another, leaving that one and returning to the first), of childhood (remembering it, celebrating it, recovering it, perpetuating it) and of religion (finding it, losing it and searching for it over and over again). But each of those themes has a more or less direct connection to the power of music and to the voice.

At one very obvious level — that of the name-checks and shout-outs — the songs are about a long list of musical styles, specific pieces of music, and the musicians who created them,

Epilogue

but the more one listens to these references in the lyrics and in the music of Morrison's songs, the more one comes to understand that these too relate to the central themes of his work. Leadbelly and Blind Lemon Jefferson might be important as musical precursors and exemplars, but they are more important still to Van the artist and Morrison the man, because he heard them 'on the street where [he] was born'. Their songs are also about the power of music. It is this power that Morrison continually — one might say ritualistically — feeds and honours in the Protestant work ethic of his relentless touring and production of albums.

And it is this power that comes across so strongly in the sound of his voice. The voice is the centre of Morrison's art and it holds very well. This is, arguably, all one needs to know. Like the child in the cradle listening to its mother's lullaby, Morrison's fans find reassurance in the singer's voice. It is a familiar sound, a sound to return to when the journeying, the questing and the day's work is done. For his audience — and, one suspects, for Morrison himself — home is where the voice is.

APPENDIX 1

DISCOGRAPHY

The Bang material

The songs Van Morrison recorded for Bert Berns in 1967 have been released many times under various titles. Broadly speaking, there are the genuine tracks and the nonsense tracks recorded in fulfilment of Morrison's contractual obligations.

BLOWIN' YOUR MIND
(1967)

- *Brown Eyed Girl* ▪ *He Ain't Give You None* ▪ *T.B. Sheets*
- *Spanish Rose* ▪ *Goodbye Baby (Baby Goodbye)*
- *Ro Ro Rosey* ▪ *Who Drove the Red Sports Car*
- *Midnight Special*

Appendix 1

THE BEST OF VAN MORRISON
(1970)

- *Spanish Rose* - *It's All Right* - *Send Your Mind* - *The Smile You Smile* - *The Back Room* - *Brown Eyed Girl* - *Goodbye Baby (Baby Goodbye)* - *Ro Ro Rosey* - *He Ain't Give You None* - *Joe Harper Saturday Morning*

T.B. SHEETS
(1974)

- *He Ain't Give You None* - *Beside You* - *It's All Right* - *Madame George* - *T.B. Sheets* - *Who Drove the Red Sports Car* - *Ro Ro Rosey* - *Brown Eyed Girl*

THIS IS WHERE I CAME IN
(1977)

- *Spanish Rose* - *Goodbye Baby (Baby Goodbye)* - *He Ain't Give You None* - *Beside You* - *Madame George* - *T.B. Sheets* - *Brown Eyed Girl* - *Send Your Mind* - *The Smile You Smile* - *The Back Room* - *Ro Ro Rosey* - *Who Drove the Red Sports Car* - *It's All Right* - *Joe Harper Saturday Morning* - *Midnight Special*

BANG MASTERS
(1991)

- *Brown Eyed Girl* - *Spanish Rose* - *Goodbye Baby (Baby Goodbye)* - *Chick A Boom* - *It's All Right* - *Send Your*

Appendix 1

Mind ▪ *The Smile You Smile* ▪ *The Back Room* ▪ *Midnight Special* ▪ *T.B. Sheets* ▪ *He Ain't Give You None* ▪ *Who Drove the Red Sports Car* ▪ *Beside You* ▪ *Joe Harper Saturday Morning* ▪ *Madame George* ▪ *Brown Eyed Girl (alternative version)* ▪ *I Love You (The Smile You Smile)*

PAYIN' DUES
(1994)

▪ *Brown Eyed Girl* ▪ *He Ain't Give You None* ▪ *T.B. Sheets* ▪ *Spanish Rose* ▪ *Goodbye Baby (Baby Goodbye)* ▪ *Ro Ro Rosey* ▪ *Who Drove the Red Sports Car* ▪ *Midnight Special* ▪ *Beside You* ▪ *It's All Right* ▪ *Madame George* ▪ *Send Your Mind* ▪ *The Smile You Smile* ▪ *The Back Room* ▪ *Joe Harper Saturday Morning* ▪ *Chick A Boom* ▪ *I Love You (The Smile You Smile)* ▪ *Brown Eyed Girl (alternative version)* ▪ *Twist and Shake* ▪ *Shake and Roll* ▪ *Stomp and Scream* ▪ *Scream and Holler* ▪ *Jump and Thump* ▪ *Drivin' Wheel* ▪ *Just Ball* ▪ *Shake it Mable* ▪ *Hold on George* ▪ *The Big Royalty Check* ▪ *Ringworm* ▪ *Savoy, Hollywood* ▪ *Freaky If You Get This Far* ▪ *Up Your Mind* ▪ *Thirty-Two* ▪ *All the Bits* ▪ *You Say France and I Whistle* ▪ *Blow in Your Nose* ▪ *Nose in Your Blow* ▪ *La Mambo* ▪ *Go for Yourself* ▪ *Want a Danish* ▪ *Here Comes Dumb George* ▪ *Chickee Coo* ▪ *Do It* ▪ *Hang on Groovy* ▪ *Goodbye George* ▪ *Dum Dum George* ▪ *Walk and Talk* ▪ *The Wooble* ▪ *Wobble and Ball*

The 'new' tracks on *Payin' Dues* first appeared on *The Lost Tapes*, issued in 1992 in Portugal, but available in many parts of the world. The same material has since resurfaced on

Appendix 1

albums entitled *Van Morrison New York Sessions '67*, *Van Morrison: The Masters* and *Brown Eyed Beginnings*. There will surely be more.

Official releases

All songs listed below are written by Morrison unless the song title is followed by a credit in square brackets. An album title in italics denotes either a Van Morrison live set or compilation, or a collaborative project.

ASTRAL WEEKS
(November 1968)

Astral Weeks

Beside You

Sweet Thing

Cyprus Avenue

The Way Young Lovers Do

Madame George

Ballerina

Slim Slow Slider

MOONDANCE
(February 1970)

And It Stoned Me

Appendix 1

Moondance

Crazy Love

Caravan

Into the Mystic

Come Running

These Dreams of You

Brand New Day

Everyone

Glad Tidings

HIS BAND AND THE STREET CHOIR

(November 1970)

Domino

Crazy Face

Give Me a Kiss

I've Been Working

Call Me Up in Dreamland

I'll Be Your Lover Too

Blue Money

Virgo Clowns

Gypsy Queen

Sweet Jannie

If I Ever Needed Someone

Street Choir

Appendix 1

TUPELO HONEY
(November 1971)

Wild Night

*(Straight to Your Heart)
Like a Cannonball*

Old Old Woodstock

Starting a New Life

You're My Woman

Tupelo Honey

*I Wanna Roo You
(Scottish Derivative)*

When That Evening Sun Goes Down

Moonshine Whiskey

SAINT DOMINIC'S PREVIEW
(August 1972)

*Jackie Wilson Said
(I'm in Heaven When You Smile)*

Gypsy

I Will Be There

Listen to the Lion

Saint Dominic's Preview

Redwood Tree

Almost Independence Day

Appendix 1

HARD NOSE THE HIGHWAY
(July 1973)

Snow in San Anselmo

Warm Love

Hard Nose the Highway

Wild Children

The Great Deception

Bein' Green [Raposo]

Autumn Song

Purple Heather [trad]

IT'S TOO LATE TO STOP NOW
(February 1974)

- *Ain't Nothin' You Can Do [Malone–Scott]* - *Warm Love* - *Into the Mystic* - *These Dreams of You* - *I Believe to My Soul [Charles]* - *I've Been Working* - *Help Me [Williamson]* - *Wild Children* - *Domino* - *I Just Want to Make Love to You [Dixon]* - *Bring it on Home to Me [Cooke]* - *Saint Dominic's Preview* - *Take Your Hands Out of My Pocket [Williamson]* - *Listen to the Lion* - *Here Comes the Night [Berns]* - *Gloria* - *Caravan* - *Cyprus Avenue*

VEEDON FLEECE
(October 1974)

Fair Play

Linden Arden Stole the Highlights

Appendix 1

Who Was That Masked Man?

Streets of Arklow

You Don't Pull No Punches, But You Don't Push the River

Bulbs

Cul de Sac

Comfort You

Come Here My Love

Country Fair

A PERIOD OF TRANSITION
(April 1977)

You Gotta Make it Through the World

It Fills You Up

The Eternal Kansas City

Joyous Sound

Flamingos Fly

Heavy Connection

Cold Wind in August

WAVELENGTH
(September 1978)

Kingdom Hall

Checkin' it Out

Natalia

Appendix 1

Venice USA

Lifetimes

Wavelength

Santa Fe [with DeShannon]/ Beautiful Obsession

Hungry For Your Love

Take it Where You Find it

INTO THE MUSIC
(August 1979)

Bright Side of the Road

Full Force Gale

Stepping Out Queen

Troubadours

Rolling Hills

You Make Me Feel So Free

Angelou

And the Healing Has Begun

It's All in the Game [Dawes–Sigman]/ You Know What They're Writing About

COMMON ONE
(August 1980)

Haunts of Ancient Peace

Summertime in England

Satisfied

Appendix 1

Wild Honey

Spirit

When Heart Is Open

BEAUTIFUL VISION
(February 1982)

Celtic Ray

Northern Muse (Solid Ground)

Dweller on the Threshold [with Murphy]

Beautiful Vision

She Gives Me Religion

Cleaning Windows

Vanlose Stairway

Aryan Mist [with Murphy]

Across the Bridge Where Angels Dwell [with Murphy]

Scandinavia (instrumental)

INARTICULATE SPEECH OF THE HEART
(March 1983)

Higher Than the World

Connswater (instrumental)

River of Time

Celtic Swing (instrumental)

Rave on, John Donne

Appendix 1

*Inarticulate Speech of the Heart No. 1
(instrumental)*

Irish Heartbeat

The Street Only Knew Your Name

Cry For Home

Inarticulate Speech of the Heart No. 2

September Night (instrumental)

LIVE AT THE GRAND OPERA HOUSE, BELFAST
(February 1984)

■ *Introduction: Into the Mystic (instrumental)/ Inarticulate Speech of the Heart* ■ *Dweller on the Threshold* ■ *It's All in the Game [Dawes–Sigman]/ You Know What They're Writing About* ■ *She Gives Me Religion* ■ *Haunts of Ancient Peace* ■ *Full Force Gale* ■ *Beautiful Vision* ■ *Vanlose Stairway* ■ *Rave On, John Donne/ Rave On, Part Two* ■ *Northern Muse (Solid Ground)* ■ *Cleaning Windows*

A SENSE OF WONDER
(December 1984)

Tore Down à la Rimbaud

Ancient of Days

Evening Meditation (instrumental)

The Master's Eyes

What Would I Do [Charles]

A Sense of Wonder

Appendix 1

Boffyflow and Spike (instrumental)

If You Only Knew [Allison]

Let the Slave (incorporating The Price of Experience) [Blake–Mitchell–Westbrook]

A New Kind of Man

NO GURU, NO METHOD, NO TEACHER
(July 1986)

Got to Go Back

Oh the Warm Feeling

Foreign Window

A Town Called Paradise

In the Garden

Tir Na Nog

Here Comes the Knight

Thanks for the Information

One Irish Rover

Ivory Tower

POETIC CHAMPIONS COMPOSE
(September 1987)

Spanish Steps (instrumental)

The Mystery

Queen of the Slipstream

I Forgot that Love Existed

Appendix 1

Sometimes I Feel Like a Motherless Child [trad]

Celtic Excavation (instrumental)

Someone Like You

Alan Watts Blues

Give Me My Rapture

Did Ye Get Healed?

Allow Me (instrumental)

IRISH HEARTBEAT

(June 1988)

with the Chieftains

■ *Star of the Country Down [trad]* ■ *Irish Heartbeat* ■ *Tá Mo Chleamhnas Déanta [trad]* ■ *Raglan Road [trad, words by Kavanagh]* ■ *She Moved Through the Fair [trad]* ■ *I'll Tell Me Ma [trad]* ■ *Carrickfergus [trad]* ■ *Celtic Ray* ■ *My Lagan Love [trad]* ■ *Marie's Wedding [trad]*

AVALON SUNSET

(June 1989)

Whenever God Shines His Light

Contacting My Angel

I'd Love to Write Another Song

Have I Told You Lately

Coney Island

I'm Tired, Joey Boy

When Will I Ever Learn to Live in God?

Appendix 1

Orangefield
Daring Night
These are the Days

THE BEST OF VAN MORRISON
(March 1990)

■ *Bright Side of the Road* ■ *Gloria* ■ *Moondance* ■ *Baby, Please Don't Go* [anon] ■ *Have I Told You Lately* ■ *Brown Eyed Girl* ■ *Sweet Thing* ■ *Warm Love* ■ *Wonderful Remark* ■ *Jackie Wilson Said (I'm in Heaven When You Smile)* ■ *Full Force Gale* ■ *And It Stoned Me* ■ *Here Comes the Night* ■ *Domino* ■ *Did Ye Get Healed?* ■ *Wild Night* ■ *Cleaning Windows* ■ *Whenever God Shines His Light* ■ *Queen of the Slipstream* ■ *Dweller on the Threshold*

ENLIGHTENMENT
(October 1990)

Real Real Gone
Enlightenment
So Quiet in Here
Avalon of the Heart
See Me Through
Youth of 1,000 Summers
In the Days Before Rock 'n' Roll [with Durcan]
Start All Over Again
She's My Baby
Memories

Appendix 1

HYMNS TO THE SILENCE
(September 1991)

Professional Jealousy

I'm Not Feeling it Anymore

Ordinary Life

Some Peace of Mind

So Complicated

I Can't Stop Loving You [Gibson]

Why Must I Always Explain?

Village Idiot

See Me Through Part II (Just a Closer Walk With Thee [anon])

Take Me Back

By His Grace

All Saints Day

Hymns to the Silence

On Hyndford Street

Be Thou My Vision [trad]

Carrying a Torch

Green Mansions

Pagan Streams

Quality Street [words by Rebennack]

It Must Be You

I Need Your Kind of Loving

Appendix 1

THE BEST OF VAN MORRISON VOLUME TWO
(January 1993)

▪ *Real Real Gone* ▪ *When Will I Ever Learn to Live in God* ▪ *Sometimes I Feel Like a Motherless Child* ▪ *In the Garden* ▪ *A Sense of Wonder* ▪ *I'll Tell Me Ma* ▪ *Coney Island* ▪ *Enlightenment* ▪ *Rave on, John Donne/ Rave on, Part Two (live)* ▪ *Don't Look Back [Hooker]* ▪ *It's All Over Now, Baby Blue [Dylan]* ▪ *One Irish Rover* ▪ *The Mystery* ▪ *Hymns to the Silence* ▪ *Evening Meditation (instrumental)*

TOO LONG IN EXILE
(June 1993)

Too Long in Exile

Big Time Operators

Lonely Avenue [Pomus]

Ball & Chain

In the Forest

Till We Get the Healing Done

Gloria

Good Morning Little Schoolgirl [Williamson]

Wasted Years

The Lonesome Road [Shilkret–Austin]

Moody's Mood for Love [Moody–Jefferson]

Close Enough for Jazz [uncredited]

Appendix 1

Before the World Was Made [Yeats–Craddock]
I'll Take Care of You [Benton]
Instrumental [Benton]
Tell Me What You Want

A NIGHT IN SAN FRANCISCO
(May 1994)

■ *Did Ye Get Healed?* ■ *It's All in the Game [Dawes–Sigman]/ Make it Real One More Time* ■ *I've Been Working* ■ *I Forgot that Love Existed* ■ *Vanlose Stairway/ Trans-Euro Train/ Fool for You [Charles]* ■ *You Make Me Feel So Free* ■ *Beautiful Vision* ■ *See Me Through/ Soldier of Fortune/ Thank You Falettinme Be Mice Elf Again [Stewart]* ■ *Ain't That Lovin' You Baby? [Hunter–Otis]* ■ *Stormy Monday [Walker]/ Have You Ever Loved a Woman? [Myles]/ No Rollin' Blues [Witherspoon]* ■ *Help Me [Williamson]* ■ *Good Morning Little Schoolgirl [Williamson]* ■ *Tupelo Honey* ■ *Moondance/ My Funny Valentine [Rodgers–Hart]*

■ *Jumpin' With Symphony Sid [Young–Beeks]* ■ *It Fills You Up* ■ *I'll Take Care of You [Benton]/ It's a Man's, Man's Man's World [Brown–Newsome]* ■ *Lonely Avenue [Pomus]/ 4 O'Clock in the Morning* ■ *So Quiet in Here/ That's Where It's At [Cooke–Alexander]* ■ *In the Garden/ You Send Me [Cooke]/ Allegheny [Staines]* ■ *Have I Told You Lately* ■ *Shakin' All Over [Kydd]/ Gloria*

Appendix 1

DAYS LIKE THIS

(June 1995)

Perfect Fit

Russian Roulette

Raincheck

You Don't Know Me [Walker–Arnold]

No Religion

Underlying Depression

Songwriter

Days Like This

I'll Never Be Free [Benjamin–Weiss]

Melancholia

Ancient Highway

In the Afternoon

HOW LONG HAS THIS BEEN GOING ON

(December 1995) with Georgie Fame

■ I Will Be There ■ The New Symphony Sid [Young–Pleasure] ■ Early in the Morning [Hickman–Jordan–Bartley] ■ Who Can I Turn To? [Newley–Bricusse] ■ Sack o' Woe [Adderley–Hendricks] ■ Moondance ■ Centrepiece [Eddison–Hendricks] ■ How Long Has This Been Going On? [G & I Gershwin] ■ Your Mind is on Vacation [Allison] ■ All Saints Day ■ Blues in the Night (My Mama Done Told Me) [Arlen–Mercer] ■ Don't Worry About a Thing [Allison] ■ That's Life [Kay–Gordon] ■ Heathrow Shuffle

Appendix 1

TELL ME SOMETHING: THE SONGS OF MOSE ALLISON
(October 1996)
with Georgie Fame, Ben Sidran and Mose Allison

[All songs by Allison] ▪ One of These Days ▪ You Can Count on Me (To Do My Part) ▪ If You Live ▪ Was ▪ Look Here ▪ City Home ▪ No Trouble Livin' ▪ Benediction ▪ Back on the Corner ▪ Tell Me Something ▪ I Don't Want Much ▪ News Nightclub ▪ Perfect Moment

THE HEALING GAME
(March 1997)

Rough God Goes Riding

Fire in the Belly

This Weight

Waiting Game

Piper at the Gates of Dawn

Burning Ground

It Once Was My Life

Sometimes We Cry

If You Love Me

The Healing Game

Appendix 1

THE PHILOSOPHER'S STONE
(June 1998)

▪ *Really Don't Know* ▪ *Ordinary People* ▪ *Wonderful Remark* ▪ *Not Supposed to Break Down* ▪ *Laughing in the Wind* ▪ *Madame Joy* ▪ *Contemplation Rose* ▪ *Don't Worry About Tomorrow* ▪ *Try For Sleep [with Platania]* ▪ *Lover's Prayer* ▪ *Twilight Zone* ▪ *Foggy Mountain Top* ▪ *Naked in the Jungle* ▪ *There There Child [with Platania]* ▪ *The Street Only Knew Your Name* ▪ *John Henry [trad]* ▪ *Western Plain [Ledbetter]* ▪ *Joyous Sound* ▪ *I Have Finally Come to Realise* ▪ *Flamingoes Fly* ▪ *Stepping Out Queen Part 2* ▪ *Bright Side of the Road* ▪ *Street Theory* ▪ *Real Real Gone* ▪ *Showbusiness* ▪ *For Mr Thomas [R Williamson]* ▪ *Crazy Jane on God [Yeats–Mathieu]* ▪ *Song of Being a Child [words by Handke]* ▪ *High Spirits*

BACK ON TOP
(March 1999)

Goin' Down Geneva

Philosopher's Stone

In the Midnight

Back on Top

When the Leaves Come Falling Down

High Summer

Reminds Me of You

New Biography

Appendix 1

Precious Time
Golden Autumn Day

THE SKIFFLE SESSIONS: LIVE IN BELFAST 1998
(January 2000)
with Lonnie Donegan and Chris Barber

- It Takes a Worried Man [trad] ▪ Lost John [trad] ▪ Goin' Home [Dvořák–Colyer] ▪ Good Morning Blues [Ledbetter] ▪ Outskirts of Town [Weldon–Jacobs] ▪ Don't You Rock Me, Daddio [trad] ▪ Alabamy Bound [trad] ▪ Midnight Special [Ledbetter] ▪ Dead or Alive [Guthrie] ▪ Frankie and Johnny [trad] ▪ Good Night Irene [Ledbetter] ▪ Railroad Bill [trad] ▪ Muleskinner Blues [Rodgers] ▪ The Ballad of Jesse James [trad] ▪ I Wanna Go Home [trad]

YOU WIN AGAIN
(September 2000)
with Linda Gail Lewis

- Let's Talk About Us [Blackwell] ▪ You Win Again [Williams] ▪ Jambalaya [Williams] ▪ Crazy Arms [Mooney–Seals] ▪ Old Black Joe [Lewis] ▪ Think Twice Before You Go [Smith] ▪ No Way Pedro ▪ A Shot of Rhythm and Blues [Thompson] ▪ Real Gone Lover [Bartholomew–Durand–Robichaux] ▪ Why Don't You Love Me [Williams] ▪ Cadillac [McDaniel] ▪ Baby (You Go What It Takes) [Otis–Stein] ▪ Boogie Chillen [Hooker–Besman]

Appendix 1

DOWN THE ROAD
(May 2002)

Down the Road

Meet Me in the Indian Summer

Steal My Heart Away

Hey Mr DJ

Talk Is Cheap

Choppin' Wood

What Makes the Irish Heart Beat

All Work and No Play

Whatever Happened to P.J. Proby?

The Beauty of the Days Gone By

Georgia on My Mind [Carmichael–Gorrell]

Only a Dream

Man Has to Struggle*

Evening Shadows [music by Bilk]

Fast Train

* included on European release only

WHAT'S WRONG WITH THIS PICTURE?
(October 2003)

What's Wrong With This Picture?

Whinin' Boy Moan

Evening in June

Appendix 1

Too Many Myths

Somerset [music by Collett–Bilk]

Meaning of Loneliness

Stop Drinking [Hopkins]

Goldfish Bowl

Once in a Blue Moon

Saint James Infirmary [trad]

Little Village

Fame

Get on with the Show

APPENDIX 2

NAME-CHECKS IN VAN MORRISON'S SONGS

Musicians

Louis Armstrong 'See Me Through Part II'
Chet Baker 'When the Leaves Come Falling Down'
Count Basie 'The Eternal Kansas City'
Sidney Bechet 'See Me Through Part II'
Big Bill Broonzy 'On Hyndford Street'
James Brown 'Real Real Gone'
Solomon Burke 'Real Real Gone'
Gene Chandler 'Real Real Gone'
Ray Charles 'These Dreams of You'
'In the Days Before Rock 'n' Roll'
'Got to Go Back'

Appendix 2

Sam Cooke 'Real Real Gone'
Claude Debussy 'On Hyndford Street'
Dr John 'Russian Roulette'
Fats Domino 'In the Days Before Rock 'n' Roll'
Billie Holiday 'The Eternal Kansas City'
John Lee Hooker 'In the Days Before Rock 'n' Roll'
Lightnin' Hopkins 'In the Days Before Rock 'n' Roll'
Mahalia Jackson 'Summertime in England'
Blind Lemon Jefferson 'Cleaning Windows'
Leadbelly 'Astral Weeks'
'Cleaning Windows'
Jerry Lee Lewis 'In the Days Before Rock 'n' Roll'
Brownie McGhee 'Cleaning Windows'
Jay McShann 'The Eternal Kansas City'
Milton 'Mezz' Mezzrow 'On Hyndford Street'
Jelly Roll Morton 'And It Stoned Me'
'On Hyndford Street'
'Whinin' Boy Moan'
Little Richard 'In the Days Before Rock 'n' Roll'
Charlie Parker 'The Eternal Kansas City'
Edith Piaf 'Saint Dominic's Preview'
Wilson Pickett 'Real Real Gone'
Elvis Presley 'In the Days Before Rock 'n' Roll'

Appendix 2

P.J. Proby 'Whatever Happened to P.J. Proby?'
Johnnie Ray 'Sometimes We Cry'
Nelson Riddle Orchestra 'Hard Nose the Highway'
Jimmie Rodgers 'Cleaning Windows'
Frank Sinatra 'Hard Nose the Highway'
Screaming Lord Sutch 'Whatever Happened to P.J. Proby?'
Sonny Terry 'Cleaning Windows'
'In the Days Before Rock 'n' Roll'
Gene Vincent 'The Street Only Knew Your Name'
Scott Walker 'Whatever Happened to P.J. Proby?'
Muddy Waters 'And the Healing Has Begun'
'Cleaning Windows'
'In the Days Before Rock 'n' Roll'
Hank Williams 'Saint Dominic's Preview'
'See Me Through Part II'
'Ancient Highway'
Sonny Boy Williamson 'Take Me Back'
Jackie Wilson 'Jackie Wilson Said (I'm in Heaven When You Smile)'
Jimmy Witherspoon 'The Eternal Kansas City'
Lester Young 'The Eternal Kansas City'

Appendix 2

Writers, philosophers, artists and actors

Samuel Beckett 'Too Long in Exile'

William Blake 'You Don't Pull No Punches, But You Don't Push the River'

'Summertime in England'

'Golden Autumn Day'

Marlon Brando 'Wild Children'

Lord Byron 'Foreign Window'

Albert Camus 'Meaning of Loneliness'

Samuel Taylor Coleridge 'Summertime in England'

Dante Alighieri 'Meaning of Loneliness'

James Dean 'Wild Children'

John Donne 'Rave on, John Donne'

T.S. Eliot 'Summertime in England'

Kahlil Gibran 'Rave on, John Donne'

Lady Gregory 'Summertime in England'

Hermann Hesse 'Meaning of Loneliness'

Christmas Humphreys 'Cleaning Windows'

James Joyce 'Summertime in England'

'Too Long in Exile'

Omar Khayyam 'Rave on, John Donne'

Jack Kerouac 'Cleaning Windows'

'On Hyndford Street'

D.H. Lawrence 'Summertime in England'

Appendix 2

Friedrich Nietzsche 'Meaning of Loneliness'
Plato 'I Forgot that Love Existed'
Edgar Allan Poe 'Fair Play'
Rembrandt van Rijn 'The Great Deception'
Arthur Rimbaud 'Tore Down à la Rimbaud'
'Foreign Window'
St John of the Cross ('Dark Night of the Soul')
'Tore Down à la Rimbaud'
'Give Me My Rapture'
Jean-Paul Sartre 'Meaning of Loneliness'
Socrates 'I Forgot that Love Existed'
Rod Steiger 'Wild Children'
Henry David Thoreau 'Fair Play'
Alan Watts 'Alan Watts Blues'
Oscar Wilde 'Fair Play'
'Too Long in Exile'
Walt Whitman 'Rave on, John Donne'
Tennessee Williams 'Wild Children'
'Contacting My Angel'
William Wordsworth 'Summertime in England'
W.B. Yeats 'Summertime in England'
'Rave on, John Donne'

BIBLIOGRAPHY

Alice Bailey, *Glamour: A World Problem*, New York: Lucis Press, 1950.

Mark W. Booth, *The Experience of Songs*, New Haven: Yale University Press, 1981

John Collis, *Van Morrison: Inarticulate Speech of the Heart*, London: Little, Brown, 1996.

Peter Conrad, *A Song of Love and Death: The Meaning of Opera*, London: Chatto & Windus, 1987.

Kenneth Grahame, *The Wind in the Willows*, London: Methuen, 1908.

Clinton Heylin, *Can You Feel the Silence? A New Biography of Van Morrison*, Chicago: Chicago Review Press, 2003.

Brian Hinton, *Celtic Crossroads: The Art of Van Morrison*, London: Sanctuary, 1997.

Patrick Humphries, *The Complete Guide to the Music of Van Morrison*, London: Omnibus, 1997.

Johnny Rogan, *Van Morrison: A Portrait of the Artist*, London: Hamish Hamilton, 1985.

Patricia Romanowski & Holly George-Warren (eds), *The New Rolling Stone Encyclopedia of Rock & Roll*, New York: Fireside/Rolling Stone Press, 1995.

Bibliography

Steve Turner, *Van Morrison: It's Too late to Stop Now*, London: Bloomsbury, 1993.

Marina Warner, *No Go the Bogeyman: Scaring, Lulling and Making Mock*, London: Chatto & Windus, 1998.

Ritchie Yorke, *Van Morrison: Into the Music*, London: Charisma, 1975.

INDEX

A & R Recording 108
'A Musical Instrument' 276
'A New Kind of Man' 205
A Night in San Francisco 12, 17, 50, 94, 96, 123, 227, 250, 261, 263, 283
A Period of Transition 11, 40, 57, 75, 162–167, 177, 201, 275
A Sense of Wonder 11, 17, 30, 66, 136, 200–205, 229, 232, 234, 311
'A Sense of Wonder' 11, 17, 30–33, 204, 274, 278
A Song of Love and Death: The Meaning of Opera 308, 314
'A Town Called Paradise' 46, 75, 83, 212, 215
'A Whiter Shade of Pale' 122
'Across the Bridge Where Angels Dwell' 192
Adams, Terry 150, 207
Ahkbar, Haji 264, 273
'Ain't Nothin' You Can Do' 42
'Alan Watts Blues' 224–226
Alcoholics Anonymous 243, 251
'All Saints Day' 251
'All the Pretty Little Horses' 306
'All Work and No Play' 293
Allair, John 178, 201, 207, 290
'Allegheny' 51
Allison, Mose 14, 201, 204, 256, 270, 272, 282, 283, 290
'Allow Me' 220
Almost Blue 125
'Almost Independence Day' 10, 126, 136, 141, 147, 236, 255, 303

American Beauty 117
American Gothic 117
'Ancient Highway' 270–271, 276
Ancient of Days 222, 244
'Ancient of Days' 201–203
'And It Stoned Me' 9, 100, 179, 235
'And the Healing Has Begun' 131, 174, 175–176, 260–261
'Angelou' 177
Annie Get Your Gun 170
Archilochus 5
Armstrong, Herbie 167, 172
Armstrong, Louis 5, 39, 174, 302
Armstrong, Neil 98
Arnold, Eddy 269
Arnold, Matthew 64, 103
'Aryan Mist' 191–192
Aspland, Robin 273
Astral Weeks 8, 9, 12, 17, 21–25, 27, 30, 33, 44, 53, 61, 65, 89, 90–98, 99, 101, 103, 105, 109, 110, 118, 122, 127, 132, 137, 146, 151, 156, 158, 167, 205, 208, 212, 215, 221, 242, 253, 257, 294, 313
'Astral Weeks' 22, 67, 92, 93, 150
'Atlantic City' 120
Atom Heart Mother 141
Atwood, Bill 140
Austin, Gene 262
'Autumn Song' 146
'Avalon of the Heart' 240, 242–243, 245
Avalon Sunset 11, 12, 55, 66, 80, 232–239, 240, 245, 250, 289

Baba, Meher 155, 207
'Baby, Please Don't Go' 7, 243
Baby Doll 35
Bacharach, Burt 83
Back on Top 13–14, 76, 77, 257, 283–288, 289, 290, 291, 297, 298, 300, 301
'Back on Top' 285, 287
Bailey, Alice 11, 185, 187–188, 190, 191, 192, 218, 236, 241, 253, 275, 276
Baker, Chet 39, 310
Ball, Kenny 28, 46
'Ball & Chain' 258–259, 264, 280
'Ballad of a Thin Man' 145, 165
'Ballerina' 96–97, 150
Band, The 99, 100, 102, 106, 109, 111, 115–116, 117, 162, 163, 167, 168, 200
Bang Records 7, 75, 92
Barber, Chris 37, 289
Bardens, Pete 168
Barrett, Elizabeth 276
Barry Lyndon 229
Basie, Count 39, 165
'Be Thou My Vision' 45, 46, 58, 247, 252
Beardsley, Aubrey 95
Beatles, The 3, 32, 34, 223, 248, 300
'Beautiful Obsession' 170
Beautiful Vision 11, 28, 60, 184–192, 197, 230, 311
'Beautiful Vision' 189
Bechet, Sidney 26, 39
'Before the World Was Made' 263
'Bein' Green' 10, 146
Bell, Derek 206, 229, 252
Bennett, Tony 126, 129, 146
Benton, Brook 263
Berlin, Irving 175
Berlin, Isaiah 5
Berliner, Jay 91, 92
Berns, Bert 7, 63, 75, 76, 79, 82, 88, 258
Berry, Chuck 254, 268
'Beside You' 44, 92–93

Bhagavad-Gita 185, 191
Bible, The 191, 202, 217
'Big Time Operators' 79, 81, 135, 258
Bilk, Acker 28, 296, 298, 301
Bill Haley and the Comets 37
Birtwistle, Harrison 5, 276
Bitches Brew 307, 313
Blackmore, Ritchie 131
Blake, William 26, 33, 46, 63, 64, 69, 70, 78, 136, 154, 179, 181, 201, 202, 205, 215, 222, 236, 243, 301, 310
Bland, Bobby 'Blue' 42, 264
Blonde on Blonde 92
Blowin' Your Mind 8, 15, 88, 111
'Blue Money' 109, 111, 113
Blue Note 81, 256, 297
'Boffyflow and Spike' 31, 205, 311, 312
'Bonaparte's Retreat' 295
'Boogie Chillen' 289
Booth, Mark W. 306
Born in Mississippi, Raised up in Tennessee 127
Born to Run 96
'Born to Run' 120
Borrow, George 103
Bradley, Liam 298
'Brand New Day' 106
Brando, Marlon 144
Branson, Richard 12, 170
Bread 117
'Bright Side of the Road' 174, 179
'Bring a Little Water, Sylvie' 37
'Bring it on Home to Me' 43
Britten, Benjamin 71
Brooks, Richard 35
Broonzy, Big Bill 39, 252
Broussard, Jules 127
'Brown Eyed Girl' 7, 88
Brown, James 39, 173, 241, 264
Brown, Johnny Mack 32
Brown, Ollie 164
Bruckner, Anton 5
Buddhism 261, 263
Buffalo Bill 116

Index

'Bulbs' 155
Bunyan, John 211
Burke, Solomon 39, 241, 286
'Burning Ground' 279–280
'Burning Love' 174
'By His Grace' 55, 251
Byrds, The 117

Cahoots 116, 121
Caledonia Soul Express 150
Caledonia Soul Orchestra 10, 43, 100, 118, 125, 139, 140, 150, 201, 207
Caledonia Studios 125, 150
'Call Me Up in Dreamland' 110, 111, 112–113, 285
Camus, Albert 301
Can You Feel the Silence? 74
'Caravan' 9, 102, 103, 142, 176
Carlyle, Thomas 61
Carmichael, Hoagy 295
Carpenter, Karen 267
'Carrickfergus' 66, 231, 249
'Carrying a Torch' 252–253
Carter, Sydney 237
'Celtic Excavation' 220
'Celtic Ray' 185–187, 231
'Celtic Swing' 196
Chandler, Gene 39, 241
Chaplin, Charlie 239
Charles, Ray 13, 27, 39, 42, 48, 105, 201, 204, 208, 214, 231, 244, 249, 256, 258, 264, 268, 290, 293, 295, 299, 300
'Checkin' it Out' 169
Chieftains Celebration 312
Chieftains, The 12, 13, 25, 31, 68, 134, 153, 183, 229–231, 247, 249–250, 252, 256, 312
'Choppin' Wood' 38, 292
Church of Ireland 215
Clannard 195
Clapton, Eric 131, 163
'Cleaning Windows' 16, 26, 60, 189–190, 252
'Close Enough for Jazz' 262

Cloud Hidden, Whereabouts Unknown: A Mountain Journal 225
Cobain, Kurt 248
Cohen, Leonard 154
'Cold Wind in August' 166
Coleridge, Samuel Taylor 63–65, 180, 310
Collis, John 15, 145, 180, 183, 219
Coltrane, John 307
Columbia Studios 119
'Come Here My Love' 157
'Come Running' 9, 104-105
'Comfortably Numb' 162
'Comfort You' 156–157
Common One 11, 47, 62, 63, 69, 104, 161, 177–184, 185, 207, 219, 220, 236, 313
Concierto de Aranjuez 312
'Coney Island' 232, 234–235
'Connswater' 195, 196
Conrad, Peter 308, 314
'Contacting My Angel' 234
Cooder, Ry 174
Cooke, Sam 39, 43, 48, 51, 153, 240, 286, 292, 303
Cooper, Tommy 26
Corvin, Donal 140
'Country Fair' 158
Costello, Elvis 5, 124
Coward, Noël 291
Cox, Mick 219
Craddock, Kenny 263
'Crazy Face' 111–112
'Crazy Jane on God' 14, 205, 283, 309
'Crazy Love' 4, 101-2, 113, 143
Credence Clearwater Revival 117
Crosby Stills Nash & Young 117
'Crossing Brooklyn Ferry' 197
Crowley, Aleister 197
Crusaders, The 163
'Cry For Home' 194, 199
'Cul De Sac' 156
Culbertson, Clive 203, 206, 233
Curved Air 177

Index

'Cyprus Avenue' 21–23, 43, 93–94, 253

Dankworth, Alec 273
'Danny Boy' 185, 209, 229
Dante Alighieri 301
'Daring Night' 237–238
David and Goliath 303
Davis, Miles 8, 91, 307, 312, 313
Davis, Richard 8, 91, 92, 94
Days Like This 13, 76, 77, 83, 265–271, 272, 298
'Days Like This' 270
Dean, James 35, 144
'Dear Lord and Father of Mankind' 46, 122
Debussy, Claude 40, 49, 252
Deep Purple 138
Delius, Frederick 87
DeShannon, Jackie 143, 149, 163, 165, 170
'Desolation Row' 84
Dexy's Midnight Runners 129
'Did Ye Get Healed?' 224, 226–227
Dixon, Willie 42, 258
Djwal Khul 187, 192
Dr. John 163, 164, 168, 254, 267, 289
'Does Your Chewing Gum Lose its Flavour on the Bedpost Overnight?' 37
'Domino' 9, 43, 109, 110, 111, 114, 119, 179, 240
Domino, Fats 244
'Don't You Rock Me, Daddio' 288
Donald, Keith 31, 298
Donegan, Lonnie 14, 37, 38, 256, 288–289
Donizetti, Gaetano 314
Donlinger, Tom 201, 207
Doonican, Val 234
Doors, The 183
'Down by the Salley Gardens' 66, 71
Down the Road 14, 28, 34, 38, 41, 47, 288–297, 298, 299, 300, 301, 302

Drifters, The 281
Drinkwater, Neil 219, 246
Drover, Martin 212, 219
'Drumshanbo Hustle' 14, 79, 135, 149
Duke Ellington Orchestra 293
Duke, Vernon 28, 282
Dulfer, Candy 259, 263, 264
Dunn, Geoff 263
Dunn, Richard 298
Durcan, Paul 244, 245
'Dweller on the Threshold' 28, 187, 188–189, 203, 279, 285
Dylan, Bob 23, 52, 56, 83, 84, 92, 93, 106, 109, 111, 117, 123, 135, 145, 163, 165, 173, 175, 187, 200, 210, 217, 226, 247, 253, 302, 307, 309, 310

Eagles, The 117
Early, Dave 233, 246
Earth Wind & Fire 164
Edwards, Ned 298
Einstein on the Beach 155
Elgar, Edward 64
Eliot, T.S. 65, 213, 282
Ellis, Pee Wee 172–173, 178, 196, 201, 207, 266, 269, 272, 284, 313
Emerson Lake and Palmer 138
Enlightenment 5, 12, 26, 40, 53, 54, 239–245, 250
'Enlightenment' 292
Enya 195
Eurovision Song Contest 13
Evans, Gil 312
'Evening in June' 300
'Evening Meditation' 203, 311, 312
'Evening Shadows' 296, 301
Everyman 181, 211
'Everyone' 106-107

'Fair Play' 150–151, 152, 153
'Fame' 76, 302–303
Fame, Georgie 13, 77, 162, 230, 232, 239, 246, 257, 266, 272, 275, 282

349

Index

'Fast Train' 296–297
Fay, Martin 229
Fields, W.C. 34
Finian's Rainbow 178
'Fire in the Belly' 67, 274–275
'Flamingos Fly' 165–166
Fleetwood Mac 169
Ford, Richard 137
'Foreign Window' 209, 210–212, 284
'4% Pantomime' 116
'Full Force Gale' 173, 174

Galway, James 229
'Georgia on My Mind' 295
Gershwin, Ira 28, 282, 309
'Get on with the Show' 303
Gibran, Khalil 196
Gibson, Don 249
Gil Evans Orchestra 307
'Give Me a Kiss' 109, 110, 112
'Give Me My Rapture' 226, 233
'Glad Tidings' 107
Glamour: A World Problem 187
Glass, Philip 154, 155
Glastonbury Festival 161
Glastonbury Tor 181
Glenn Miller Orchestra 36
'Gloria' 7, 41, 43, 79, 255, 261, 264, 280, 283
'Goin' Down Geneva' 284
'Golden Autumn Day' 77–78, 287, 291, 301
Golden Dawn, Hermetic Order of the 194, 197
'Goldfish Bowl' 76, 80–82, 301–302
'Good Morning Little Schoolgirl' 94, 261, 263
Goodall, Lee 290, 298
Goodman, Benny 5
'Got to Go Back' 27, 29, 208, 209
'Gotta Get You Off My Mind' 286
Gould, Glenn 3
Grahame, Kenneth 71–72, 276–279
Grateful Dead, The 117
Green, Leo 272

Green, Mick 284, 289, 298
'Green Mansions' 253
Gregory, Steve 246
Grey, Zane 90
Griffin, Colin 290
Guida, Carol 149, 157
Guthrie, Woody 289
'Gypsy' 129, 136
'Gypsy Queen' 110, 113

Hammerstein, Oscar 28
Hard Nose the Highway 10, 75, 79, 138–148, 149, 172
'Hard Nose the Highway' 143–144
Hardy, Thomas 180–181
Harrison, George 37, 95
'Haunts of Ancient Peace' 69, 178, 181–182
'Have I Told You Lately' 224, 232, 234, 239
'Have You Ever Loved a Woman?' 6
Haydn, Josef 5
Hayes, David 140, 150, 173, 201, 207, 289, 298
'Heartbreak Hotel' 35
'Heathrow Shuttle' 272
'Heavy Connection' 166
Helm, Levon 163, 230
Henderson, Marlo 164
Hendrix, Jimi 98, 127
'Here Comes the Knight' 216
'Here Comes the Night' 4, 7, 88
Hergest Ridge 180
Hesse, Hermann 301
'Hey Mister Mr DJ' 291–292
Heylin, Clinton 15, 74, 118, 220, 249
'High Summer' 285
'Higher Than the World' 195, 196
Hinton, Brian 15, 220
His Band and the Street Choir 9, 43, 107, 108-115, 116, 120–121, 123, 143, 147
'Hit the Road Jack' 293
Ho Chi Minh 140
Holiday, Billie 39, 165

350

Index

Holland, Matt 284, 289, 298
Holly, Buddy 281
Holmes Brothers, The 256
Holst, Gustav 71
Holy Grail 154, 198, 213, 240, 242
'Hoochie Coochie Man' 41
Hooker, John Lee 13, 39, 41, 44, 49, 127, 137, 162, 169, 244, 255, 256, 261, 281, 283, 289
Hopkins, Lightnin' 38, 81, 244, 301
'House of the Risin' Sun' 113
Houston, Cissy 102
'How Are Things in Glocca Morra?' 178
'How Do You Sleep?' 135
How Long Has This Been Going On 14, 81, 101, 272, 273, 283
'How Long Has This Been Going On?' 309
Howerd, Frankie 26
Hubbard, L. Ron 55, 194, 207
Hudson, Garth 168, 169
Humphreys, Christmas 26, 190, 260
Humphries, Patrick 179, 219, 249
'Hungry For Your Love' 170
Hurley, Pete 289, 298
Hymns to the Silence 12, 17, 29, 46, 53, 55, 58, 59, 62, 70, 76, 118, 151, 246–254, 256, 257, 285
'Hymns to the Silence' 251

'I Believe to my Soul' 27, 42, 295
'(I Can't Get No) Satisfaction' 182
'I Can't Get Started' 28
'I Can't Stop Loving You' 249
'I Cover the Waterfront' 44–45, 137
'I Forgot that Love Existed' 223
'I Just Want to Make Love to You' 42, 258
'I Need Your Kind of Loving' 254
'I Shall Be Released' 106, 163
'I Wanna Roo You' 117, 118, 123

'I Will Be There' 130
'I'd Love to Write Another Song' 80, 234
'I'll Be Your Lover Too' 109, 113
'I'll Never be Free' 270
'I'll Take Care of You' 263–264
'I'll Tell Me Ma' 25, 229, 231
'I'm in the Mood for Love' 262
'I'm Not Feeling it Anymore' 76, 248
'I'm Tired, Joey Boy' 235–236
'I've Been Working' 43, 109, 110, 112
'If I Ever Needed Someone' 109, 114
'If You Love Me' 281–282
'If You Only Knew' 204
'If You See Her Say Hello' 84
'In a Silent Way' 313
'In the Afternoon' 271
'In the days before rock 'n' roll' 26, 196, 243–245
'In the Forest' 259, 260, 264, 278, 280
'In the Garden' 11, 17, 50–51, 53, 96, 124, 212–215, 278
'In the Midnight' 284
'In the Mood' 36
Inarticulate Speech of the Heart 11, 56, 186, 193–200, 203, 219, 220, 230, 232, 311, 312
'Inarticulate Speech of the Heart No. 1.' 311
'Inarticulate Speech of the Heart No.2.' 199
Incredible String Band 194
'Independence Day' 137
'Intimations of Immortality' 214
Into the Music 11, 22, 68, 114, 131, 172–177, 178, 183, 184, 206, 228, 255, 260, 269
'Into the Mystic' 103–104, 242
Irish Heartbeat 12, 15, 25, 68, 159, 177, 187, 224, 227–231, 232, 238, 249, 313
'Irish Heartbeat' 198
Irwin, Bobby 289, 298

Index

Isham, Mark 69, 173, 178, 201, 313
'Isis' 84
'It Fills You Up' 165, 166
'It Must Be You' 254
'It Once Was My Life' 28, 281
'It's a Man's, Man's, Man's World' 264
It's Too Late to Stop Now 10, 42, 43, 102, 130, 144, 147, 150, 257, 258, 283, 298, 309, 314
'It's All in the Game' 174
'Ivory Tower' 209, 218

Jack Johnson 307
'Jackie Wilson Said (I'm in heaven when you smile)' 10, 128–129, 179
Jackson, Mahalia 39, 65, 179
Jackson, Michael 307
James, Harry 300
James, Jesse 112
Jason and the Argonauts 154
Jefferson, Blind Lemon 26, 39, 190, 315
Jehovah's Witnesses 48, 52, 57–58, 59, 168, 207, 221, 241
'Jerusalem' 46, 215, 243
Jesus Christ 64, 179, 237, 243, 261
Jesus Christ Superstar 139
Jethro Tull 138
John Aldiss Choir 141
John Wesley Harding 111, 117
Johnson, Ronnie 239–240, 263
Jones, Booker T. 44
Jones, Brian 98
Jones, Tom 13, 252–253, 281
Joplin, Janis 98, 127
Jordan, Mark 119, 127, 173
Joseph of Arimathea 64, 236, 243
Jones, Rufus Matthew 62
Joyce, James 33, 87
'Joyous Sound' 165
'Jump and Thump' 75
Jung, Carl Gustav 34
'Jungleland' 96
'Just a Closer Walk with Thee' 45, 247, 250

Kavanagh, Patrick 70, 231
Kay, Connie 8, 9, 91, 93, 118–119, 127
Kazan, Elia 35
Keen, Sam 274
Kennedy, Brian 51, 123, 230, 266, 267, 270, 275, 284
'Kentucky Avenue' 95
Kenyon, Carol 201, 233, 246
Kermit the Frog 10, 146
Kerouac, Jack 16, 26, 190, 252
Khayyam, Omar 196
King, B.B. 13, 256, 281
King's Hotel, Newport 248
Kingdom Hall 55, 57, 168, 221, 227
'Kingdom Hall' 57, 168, 172, 285
Kissoon, Katie 172, 201, 233, 246, 273
Klingberg, John 100, 108
Knopfler, Mark 13, 125, 190
Konitz, Lee 311
Krishna 185, 192, 241
Krishnamurti 207
Kubrik, Stanley 229
'Kumbaya' 106

Labes, Jeff 100, 102, 106, 118, 140, 150, 207
Lauper, Cyndi 307
Lavengro 103
Leadbelly 26, 37, 38, 40–41, 105, 190, 289, 290, 315
Led Zeppelin 181
Lemmon, Jack 243
Lennon, John 5, 37, 135, 266, 270, 310
'Let the Slave' 205
Lewis, Jerry Lee 244, 289
Lewis, Linda Gayle 14, 289, 290, 298
'Lifetimes' 168
'Like a Cannonball' 117, 120–121
'Like a Rolling Stone' 84
'Linden Arden Stole the Highlights' 112, 152

Index

'Listen to the Lion' 10, 43–44, 96, 124, 130–133, 134, 136, 247, 314
Little Richard 35, 244
'Little Sister' 258
'Little Village' 302
Live at the Grand Opera House, Belfast 11, 103, 191, 200–201, 310
Lomax, Alan 299
'Lonely Avenue' 258, 262, 263–264
Lord of the Dance 237–238
Loughborough University 206, 226
Lovano, Joe 311
Lucia di Lammermoor 314
Lyle, Tina 263
Lytle, Foggy 298

'Madame George' 17, 21–24, 53, 92, 95–96, 97, 120, 150
Mahler, Gustav 1, 5, 6, 25
Malabar, Gary 100, 118–119, 127, 134, 140, 190
'Man Has to Struggle' 296
'Mannish Boy' 41
Manuel, Richard 116, 305
Manx, Harry 136
Marcus, Greil 23
Marcus, Tony 172, 178
'Marie's Wedding' 231
Marley, Bob 128
Mathieu, William 205
McBride, Reggie 164
McCartney, Paul 37, 151, 310
McCormack, John 228, 231, 234
McFee, John 119, 123, 127
McGhee, Brownie 26, 37
McGlynn, Arty 193, 233, 268
McLean, Jackie 81
McShann, Jay 39, 165
'Meaning of Loneliness' 301
Meet Me in St Louis 29
'Meet Me in the Indian Summer' 291, 293
'Melancholia' 265, 270
'Memories' 245
'Memphis Tennessee' 254

Mercury Records 172, 201
Merenstein, Lewis 91, 97, 105, 164, 242
Messenger, Doug 127
Messiaen, Olivier 5
Mezzrow, Milton 'Mez' 39, 252
Michie, Chris 185, 201, 207
Miller, Edward 47
Mingus, Charlie 81
Mister Lucky 44
Mitchell, Adrian 204
Mitchell, Joni 163, 310
Mix, Tom 32
Modern Jazz Quartet 8, 91
Moloney, Paddy 58, 229, 279
Monarchs, the 7, 264
Monk, Thelonious 5, 81
Montreux Jazz Festival 149, 155, 168
Montrose, Ronnie 119, 127, 142, 149
Moody Blues, The 138
Moody, James 262
Moondance 9, 98–107, 109, 110, 137, 143, 295
'Moondance' 9, 83, 101, 166, 283
'Moonshine Whiskey' 124
Morrison, George 6, 38, 228
Morrison, Jim 96, 127
Morrison, Shana 13, 111, 228, 269, 270, 281
Morrison, Van
 – and Caledonian culture 118, 125–126, 133, 147, 148, 250
 – and concept of a 'ray' 186
 – and 'glamour' 187–188, 192, 218
 – and music therapy 206
 – and the 'burning ground' 188
 – and the 'Troubles' 70, 293
 – as an agnostic 189
 – complaint songs 73–84
 – dubbed 'The Belfast Cowboy' 116
 – early Musical experiences 6–7
 – expatriation 87–90

Index

– fascination with Wild West 116–117, 151–152, 170
– flirtation with Scientology 194
– his voice 4–5, 305–315
– influence of Protestantism 58–60
– influence on Bruce Springsteen 93, 96, 120, 128–129, 137, 253
– move toward 'easy listening' music 224
– musical heroes 34–49
– relations with media 2
– repeated patterns of creative behaviour 16
– return to Ireland 10, 12
– songs about childhood 21–33
– songs inspired by nature and literature 60–72
– songs of transcendence and religion 50–60

Morrison, Violet 6, 45, 48, 57–58, 213, 228, 231
Morton, Jelly Roll 39, 252, 299
Moving Hearts 31, 201, 229, 311
Mozart, Wolfgang Amadeus 314
Muleskinner Blues 289
Mulligan, Gerry 81
Munch, Ulla 190, 212
Muscle Shoals Sound Studios 173
Music from Big Pink 100
Music: Its Secret Influences Through the Ages 11
'My Back Pages' 93
'My Lagan Love' 231
'My Old Man's a Dustman' 37

Naftalin, Mark 127
Napoleon 303
Nashville Skyline 117
'Natalia' 169, 172
Nelson Riddle Orchestra 40, 143
Nero 303
Never Get Out of These Blues Alive 127
Newman, Randy 83
'New Biography' 76, 286

New York Post 35
Nietzsche, Friedrich 301
No Guru, No Method, No Teacher 11, 17, 27, 46, 61, 62, 76, 96, 97, 161, 179, 182, 189, 192, 206–218, 220, 222, 223, 224, 227, 232, 234, 236, 241, 244, 248, 257, 284, 286
No Reason to Cry 163
'No Religion' 269
'No Rollin' Blues' 6
'No Way, Pedro' 289
'Nobody Told Me' 266
'Non, je ne regrette rien' 134
'Northern Muse (Solid Ground)' 187

O'Connor, Sinead 186
Oakland Symphony Orchestra 141
Ofarim, Esther and Abi 262
'Oh the Warm Feeling' 209–210
'Oil and Blood' 213
'Ol' Man River' 249
'Old Old Woodstock' 121
Oldfield, Mike 180
'On Hyndford street' 17, 29, 33, 40, 53, 62, 151, 198, 247, 251–252
On the Road 190
On the Waterfront 144
'Once in a Blue Moon' 302
'One Irish Rover' 218
'Only a Dream' 295–296
'Orangefield' 232, 237
'Ordinary Life' 248–249, 253, 259
'Out of the Cradle Endlessly Rocking' 208

Pacific High Recording Studios 119, 127
'Pagan Streams' 253
Page, Jimmy 131
Pan 276
Panic 276
Paradise Lost 285
Paramount Jazz Band 28, 296
Parker, Alan 111

Index

Parker, Charlie 39, 165
Parry, Hubert 46
Payin' Dues 75
Payne, John 8, 91, 97
Pearce, Steve 219, 246
'Perfect Fit' 267, 302
Perkins, Carl 256
Philosopher's Stone 221
'Philosopher's Stone' 284, 287, 300
Piaf, Edith 40, 49, 134
Pickett, Wilson 39, 109, 112, 114, 146, 153, 241
Pierrot, Lunaire 5
Piggott, Lester 244
Pink Floyd 138, 141, 276
'Piper at the Gates of Dawn' 71, 276–279
Planet, Janet 8, 9, 10, 46, 108, 113, 116, 117, 118, 137, 265
Platania, John 42, 100, 108, 111, 113, 118–119, 140, 207
Plato 187, 211, 223
Poe, Edgar Allan 151
Poetic Champions Compose 11, 67, 158, 219–227, 232, 233, 234, 257, 311, 312
Pogues, The 186
Pointer Sisters, The 164
Polydor Records 233, 289
Pomus, Doc 258
Pope John Paul II 229
'Positively 4th Street' 135
Povey, Gavin 298
'Precious Time' 286–287
Prelude to the Genesis 262
Presley, Elvis 35, 57, 174, 244, 249
Proby, P.J. 293–294
Procol Harum 122, 138
'Professional Jealousy' 55, 70, 76, 247–248
Prophet, Elizabeth Clare 175
Psalm 69 202–203
'Purple Heather' 147

'Quality Street' 254
Quarry Men, The 37
'Queen of the Slipstream' 221–223

Radio Luxembourg 29, 40, 244
'Raglan Road' 231
'Raincheck' 76, 83, 265, 267–268
Raposo, Joe 146
'Rave on, John Donne' 114, 194, 195, 196–197, 198, 310
Ray, Johnnie 281
Ray, Nicholas 35
'Real Real Gone' 39–40, 240–241, 243
Rebel Without a Cause 35
Rebennack, Mac 164
Record Plant 163, 165, 172, 173
Red Norbo Quartet 270
Redding, Otis 112
'Redwood Tree' 135–136
Reed, Lou 310
'Reet Petite' 128
Reload 281
'Reminds Me of You' 286
Richard, Cliff 13, 55, 162, 226, 232, 233, 239
Rimbaud, Arthur 26, 202
'River of Time' 195–196, 197
Robertson, Robbie 106, 121, 238
Robeson, Paul 262
Robinson, Smokey 4
Rocca, Michelle 13, 265–266, 274
'Rock Around the Clock' 35
'Rock Island Line' 37
'Rock-a-bye Baby' 306
'Rockingham' 47
Rodgers, Jimmie 16, 38, 289
Rodgers, Richard 28
Rodrigo, Joaquín 312
Rogan, Johnnie 14–15
'Rolling Hills' 173, 177, 178, 184, 228
Rolling Stones, The 42, 115, 163, 164, 182
Rosicrucians 26, 194, 207, 241
Rothermel, Jim 155
'Rough God Goes Riding' 273–274
Rubin, Nathan 140, 150
'Russian Roulette' 265, 267

Index

'Sad-eyed Lady of the Lowlands' 92
Sailing to Philadelphia 125
Saint Dominic's Preview 9, 43, 96, 124, 125–138, 139, 143, 146, 147, 148, 150, 167, 314
'Saint Dominic's Preview' 43, 133–135
'Saint James Infirmary' 302
St John, Kate 208, 257, 259, 270
Salisbury 141
Salisbury, Tom 133
Salmins, Ralph 273
Sample, Joe 163
Samson and Delilah 303
'Santa Fe' 170
Sartre, Jean-Paul 301
'Satisfaction' 182
'Satisfied' 182
Savannah, John 263
'Save the Last Dance for Me' 258
'Scandinavia' 190, 192, 196, 311
Schlosser, Rick 119, 127, 129, 140
Schoenberg, Arnold 5, 262
Schroer, Jack 100, 108, 118, 127, 128, 140, 150
Scientology 11, 55, 162, 194, 195, 241
Scorsese, Martin 102, 163, 238
Scott, Cyril 11, 175
Scott, Johnny 298
Scott, Nicky 247, 257, 263, 289, 298
Scott, Ronnie 53, 272, 309
'Scream and Holler' 75
'See Me Through' 243, 251
'See Me Through Part 2' 247, 250
'Send in the Clowns' 310
Sgt Pepper's Lonely Hearts Club Band 32, 34, 300
'September Night' 312
Shaar, Dahaud 108, 113, 118, 140, 150
'Shake and Roll' 75
Shakespeare, William 188
Shaw, David 108
'She Gives Me Religion' 189, 191
'She Moved Through the Fair' 231, 313
'She's My Baby' 245
Shepherds of the Delectable Mountains 141
Shilkret, Nathaniel 262
Shorter, Wayne 307
Sidran, Ben 272
Sinatra, Frank 35, 39, 126, 129, 132, 143, 146, 262
Sketches of Spain 312
'Slane' 58
Sledge, Percy 112
Slim Slow Slider 8–9, 97, 303
Slow Train Coming 173
Smith, Warren 91
'Snow in San Anselmo' 10, 141–143, 166
'So Complicated' 249
'So quiet in here' 5, 53, 240, 241–242
Socrates 223
'Some Peace of Mind' 249
'Someone Like You' 224
'Somerset' 28, 301
'Sometimes I Feel Like a Motherless Child' 223
'Sometimes We Cry' 281
Sondheim, Stephen 310
Songs of Praise 46
'Songwriter' 76, 80, 83, 265, 269–270
'Spanish Steps' 220, 312
Spillane, Davy 31, 193
'Spirit' 183
Sprechstimme 5
Springer, Rob 140
Springsteen, Bruce 6, 93, 96, 120, 124, 128, 137, 253
'Star of the County Down' 228, 231
Starr, Kay 295
'Start All Over Again' 245
'Starting a New Life' 115, 121
'Steal My Heart Away' 291
Steiger, Rod 144
'Stepping Out Queen' 173–174, 177, 269
Stewart, Rod 232, 234, 239

Index

Stockhausen, Karlheinz 34
Stomp and Scream' 75
Stone Alone 163
Stonehenge 179
'Stop Drinking' 81, 301
'Stormy Monday' 6
'(Straight to Your Heart) Like a Cannonball' See 'Like a Cannonball'
'Stranger on the Shore' 28–29
Stravinsky, Igor 5
'Street Choir' 109, 114
'Streets of Arklow' 150, 152–153
'Summer Set' 28
'Summertime in England' 47, 63–65, 124, 179–180, 196, 313
'Sweet Bird of Youth' 244
'Sweet Jannie' 109, 110, 114
'Sweet Sixteen' 143
'Sweet Thing' 93, 100, 213
Sweetheart of the Rodeo 117
Synge, John Millington 68

'T.B. Sheets' 44, 88, 214
'Tá Mo Chleamhnas Déanta' 231
'Take it Where You Find it' 170–171
'Take Me Back' 250–251
'Take Your Hands Out of My Pocket' 43
'Talk is Cheap' 41, 292
'Tangled Up in Blue' 84
Tell Me Something 14, 81, 272, 273, 282, 283
'Tell Me What You Want' 263
Templeman, Ted 119, 128, 140, 164
Tennyson, Alfred Lord 15
Terry, Sonny 26, 37, 41, 244
'Thanks for the Information' 217, 224
'The Beauty of the Days Gone By' 47, 294–295
The Blackboard Jungle 35
The Commitments 111
'The Dharma Bums' 16, 190

'The End' 183
'The Eternal Kansas City' 40, 165, 166, 275
The Experience of Songs 306
The Female Eunuch 122
The Gods Await 280
'The Great Deception' 75, 145
The Healing Game 11, 13, 28, 67, 71, 175, 188, 256, 257, 272–282, 283, 284, 289, 291, 297
'The Healing Game' 282
The King and I 28
The King of Comedy 238
The Lark Ascending 139
The Last Waltz 102, 167
'The Lonesome Road' 262, 295
The Magic Flute 314
'The March of the Siamese Children' 28, 46
'The Master's Eyes' 203–204, 205
'The Mystery' 158, 220, 227, 233
The Philosopher's Stone 14, 24, 79, 149, 163, 205, 283
'The Prelude' 63, 65
'The Price of Experience' 205
The Return of the Native 180
'The Scholar Gipsy' 64, 103
'The Second Coming' 314
The Skiffle Sessions 14, 37, 288–289, 298
The Smoker You Get, the Player You Drink 153
'The Street Only Knew Your Name' 195, 198
'The Times They Are A-Changin''
'The Trolley Song' 29
The Wall 161–162
'The Waste Land' 213
'The Way Young Lovers Do' 94–95
'The Weight' 106
The Wind in the Willows 71–72, 276–279
Them 4, 7, 79, 88, 168, 189, 191, 216, 224, 243, 261, 264
'These are the Days' 238, 245
'These Dreams of You' 105, 285

Index

Theosophy 11, 194, 241, 276, 280
'Things Ain't What They Used to Be' 293
'This Weight' 275
Thoreau, Henry David 151
Thornton, Bianca 201
'Thunder Road' 96
'Till We Get the Healing Done' 260–261, 264
Tilton, Colin 101
Tingley, Katherine 280
'Tir Na Nog' 215–216
Tolkein, J.R.R. 70
Tommy 139
'Tomorrow Shall Be My Dancing Day' 237
Too Long in Exile 12, 76, 79, 256–264, 265, 271, 272, 280, 283, 284, 289, 295
'Too Long in Exile' 257–258
'Too Many Myths' 301
'Tore Down à la Rimbaud' 201, 202, 204, 234
Townhouse Studios 207
Trench, Fiachra 219, 242, 246, 284, 287, 289, 298
Tropea, John 150
'Troubadours' 177
Tupelo Honey 9, 69, 115–125, 143, 147, 149, 245, 249, 253, 265
'Tupelo Honey' 46, 118, 122–123, 234
Turner, Steve 15
'Twist and Shake' 75

U2 56, 186
Ulysses 33, 87
'Under Ben Bulben' 216
'Underlying Depression' 77, 265, 269
Uriah Heep 141

Valli, Frankie 284
van Hooke, Peter 168, 201, 207
Vanlose Stairway 190–191
Vaughan Williams, Ralph 64, 70–71, 139, 141, 180

Veedon Fleece 10–11, 62, 89, 104, 112, 132, 147, 148–159, 162, 168, 170, 177, 184, 200, 210, 228, 251
'Venice USA' 169
Verve 81, 272
'Village Idiot' 249–250
Vincent, Gene 199
Virgin Records 289
'Virgo Clowns' 113

Waites, Tom 4, 95
'Waiting Game' 275–276, 279
Walker, Cindy 269
Wall, Max 26
Wally Heider Recording 119
Walsh, Joe 153
'Warm Love' 143
Warner Bros. 8, 162, 167, 172
Warner, Marina 306
'Wasted Years' 261
Waters, Muddy 26, 39, 41, 49, 163, 176, 244
Waters, Roger 161
Watkins, Geraint 284, 289
Watts, Alan 26, 224–226
Watts, Isaac 47,
Wavelength 11, 57, 114, 167–172, 177, 221, 265
'Wavelength' 169–170
Wells, Junior 13
Wesley, Charles 47
Westbrook, Mike 204
'What Makes the Irish Heart Beat' 292–293
'What Would I Do' 204
What's Wrong With This Picture? 14, 17, 28, 76, 81, 247, 256, 297–303
'What's Wrong With This Picture?' 300
'Whatever Happened to P.J. Proby?' 293–294
'When Heart Is Open' 183–184, 278, 303, 313–314
'When I Survey the Wondrous Cross' 47

Index

'When That Evening Sun Goes Down' 123
'When the Leaves Come Tumbling Down' 285
'When Will I Ever Learn to Live in God?' 236
'Whenever God Shines His Light' 55, 232, 233–234, 239
'Whinin' Boy Moan' 299–300
Whitman, Walt 93, 94, 106, 117, 196–197, 202, 208, 210
Whittier, John G. 46
'Who Was That Masked Man' 112, 152
'Why Must I Always Explain' 55, 60, 66, 76, 80, 118, 131, 249
Wickett, Alan 'Sticky' 298
'Wild Children' 144
'Wild Honey' 182
'Wild Mountain Thyme' 147
'Wild Night' 9, 119–120, 179, 240
Wilde, Oscar 151
Williams, Hank 26, 37, 135, 289, 290
Williams, Tennessee 144, 234, 244
Williamson, Robin 177, 194, 206
Williamson, Sonny Boy 39, 42, 43, 48, 251, 261
Wilson, Jackie 39, 128
Windham Hill 195
Windmill Lane Studios 266, 273, 284
Winning, Martin 298
Wisdom, Norman 26
Wisseloord Studios 149
Witherspoon, Jimmy 13, 39, 165

'Wonderful Remark' 149, 238
'Wonderful World' 292
Wood, Grant 117
Woodstock 9, 88, 115–116
Wool Hall Studios 219, 257, 272, 284, 289, 298
Wordsworth, William 63–65, 180, 214, 310
Worth, Harry 26
Wrekin Trust 206, 226
Wyman, Bill 163

Yeats, W.B. 13, 14, 68, 69, 163, 196–197, 205, 213, 216, 262–263, 309, 310, 314
Yes 138
York, Ritchie 14
'You Don't Know Me' 268–269
'You Don't Pull No Punches, But You Don't Push the River' 153–155, 270
'You Gotta Make it Through the World' 75, 164
'You Know What They're Writing About' 174, 303
'You Make Me Feel So Free' 174
'You Send Me' 51
You Win Again 14, 288–289, 298
'You're My Woman' 121–122
Young, Lester 39, 165
Young, Neil 163
'Youth of 1,000 Summers' 240, 244
'Youngblood' 258

'Zen Buddhism' 26, 225, 241, 260, 292

ACKNOWLEDGMENTS

The authors would like to thank Mark W. Booth for permission to quote from his book, *The Experience of Songs*, and Peter Conrad for permission to quote from *A Song of Love and Death*. At ABC Books, Jacqueline Kent commissioned this volume, Jo Mackay saw it through and Jon Gibbs edited it with a rare degree of passion for its contents. Thanks to them all. Andrew Ford would like to apologise to his wife, Anni Heino, for the sheer volume (in both senses) of Van Morrison's music to which she has recently been subjected. He also offers belated thanks to his friends Diana Wood and Graham Devlin who 'in another time, in another place' first introduced him to Van Morrison and his songs. Martin Buzacott would like to thank Monica Wittenberg for her support during the research and writing of the book, and Daniel Buzacott for his assistance in the preparation of the index.